100 CASES
in Surgery

James A Gossage MBBS BSc MRCS
Specialist Registrar in General Surgery

Bijan Modarai MBBS BSc PhD MRCS
Specialist Registrar in General Surgery

Arun Sahai MBBS BSc MRCS
Specialist Registrar in Urology

Richard Worth MBBS BSc MRCS
Orthopaedic Research Fellow

Volume Editor:
Kevin G Burnand MS FRCS
Professor of Vascular Surgery, Academic Department of Surgery, King's College London School of Medicine at Guy's, King's and St Thomas' Hospitals, London, UK

100 Cases Series Editor:
P John Rees MD FRCP
Dean of Medical Undergraduate Education, King's College London School of Medicine at Guy's, King's and St Thomas' Hospitals, London, UK

Hodder Arnold

A MEMBER OF THE HODDER HEADLINE GROUP

First published in Great Britain in 2008 by
Hodder Arnold, an imprint of Hodder Education and a member of the Hodder Headline Group,
An Hachette Livre UK Company, 338 Euston Road, London NW1 3BH

http://www.hoddereducation.com

Hodder Headline's policy is to use papers that are natural, renewable and recyclable products and made from wood grown in sustainable forests. The logging and manufacturing processes are expected to conform to the environmental regulations of the country of origin.

Whilst the advice and information in this book are believed to be true and accurate at the date of going to press, neither the author[s] nor the publisher can accept any legal responsibility or liability for any errors or omissions that may be made. In particular, (but without limiting the generality of the preceding disclaimer) every effort has been made to check drug dosages; however it is still possible that errors have been missed. Furthermore, dosage schedules are constantly being revised and new side-effects recognized. For these reasons the reader is strongly urged to consult the drug companies' printed instructions before administering any of the drugs recommended in this book.

British Library Cataloguing in Publication Data
A catalogue record for this book is available from the British Library

Library of Congress Cataloging-in-Publication Data
A catalog record for this book is available from the Library of Congress

ISBN 978 0 340 94170 6

1 2 3 4 5 6 7 8 9 10

Commissioning Editor: Sara Purdy
Project Editor: Jane Tod
Production Controller: Lindsay Smith
Cover Design: Laura DeGrasse
Indexer: Laurence Errington

Typeset in 10/12 RotisSerif by Charon Tec Ltd (A Macmillan Company), Chennai, India
www.charontec.com
Printed and bound in Spain

CONTENTS

PREFACE

We hope this book will give a good introduction to common surgical conditions seen in everyday surgical practice. Each question has been followed up with a brief overview of the condition and its immediate management. The book should act as an essential revision aid for surgical finals and as a basis for practising surgery after qualification.

I would like to thank my co-authors for all their help and expertise in each of the surgical specialties. I would also like to thank the following people for their help with illustrations: Professor KG Burnand, Mr MJ Forshaw, Mr M Reid and Mr A Liebenberg.

James A Gossage
October 2007

ABBREVIATIONS

ABPI ankle–brachial pressure index
ACTH adrenocorticotrophic hormone
ALP alkaline phosphatase
AP anterior-posterior
APTT activated partial thromboplastin time
ASA American Society of Anaesthesiologists
AST aspartate transaminase
ATLS Advanced Trauma and Life Support
BMI body mass index
BNF *British National Formulary*
BPH benign prostatic hyperplasia
CBD common bile duct
CEA carcinoembryonic antigen
CGT gamma-glutamyl transferase
COPD chronic obstructive pulmonary disease
CRP C-reactive protein
CSDH chronic subdural haematoma
CT computerized tomography
DVT deep vein thrombosis
ECG electrocardiogram
EMG electromyogram
ENT ear, nose and throat
ERCP endoscopic retrograde cholangiopancreatography
ESR erythrocyte sedimentation rate
EUA examination under anaesthesia
FAST focused abdominal sonographic technique
FEV_1 forced expiratory volume in one second
FNAC fine needle aspiration cytology
FVC forced vital capacity
GCS Glasgow Coma Score
GGT gamma-glutamyl transferase
GP general practitioner
Hb haemoglobin
HbS haemoglobin S
HCG human chorionic gonadotrophin
HDU high-dependency unit
HiB Haemophilus influenzae type B
ICU intensive care unit
IgA immunoglobulin A
INR international normalized ratio
IPSS International Prostate Symptom Score
IVU intravenous urethrogram

KUB	kidney, ureter, bladder
LDH	lactate dehydrogenase
LUTS	lower urinary tract symptoms
MEN	multiple endocrine neoplasia
MRCP	magnetic resonance cholangiopancreatography
MRI	magnetic resonance imaging
NAD	no abnormality detected
NEXUS	National Emergency X-Radiography Utilization Group
NSAID	non-steroidal anti-inflammatory drug
NSGCT	non-seminomatous germ cell tumour
OGD	oesophagogastroduodenoscopy
pco_2	partial pressure of carbon dioxide
PE	pulmonary embolism
po_2	partial pressure of oxygen
PSA	prostate-specific antigen
PTH	parathyroid hormone
T_3	tri-iodothyronine
T_4	thyroxine
TIA	transient ischaemic attack
TSH	thyroid-stimulating hormone
TURBT	transurethral resection of a bladder tumour
TURP	transurethral resection of the prostate
UMN	upper motor neurone
$\dot{V}/\dot{Q}$	ventilation–perfusion ratio
WCC	white cell count

GENERAL AND COLORECTAL

CASE 1: A LUMP IN THE GROIN

History

A 51-year-old woman presents to the emergency department with a painful right groin. She also has some lower abdominal distension and has vomited twice on the way to the hospital. She has passed some flatus but has not opened her bowels since yesterday. She is otherwise fit and well and is a non-smoker. She lives with her husband and four children.

Examination

On examination she looks unwell. Her blood pressure is 106/70 mmHg and the pulse rate is 108/min. She is febrile with a temperature of 38.0°C. The abdomen is tender, particularly in the right iliac fossa, and there is lower abdominal distension. There is a small swelling in the right groin which is originating below and lateral to the pubic tubercle. The lump is irreducible and no cough impulse is present. Digital rectal examination is unremarkable and bowel sounds are hyperactive.

INVESTIGATIONS

		Normal
Haemoglobin	14.1 g/dL	11.5–16.0 g/dL
White cell count	18.0×10^9/L	$4.0–11.0 \times 10^9$/L
Platelets	361×10^9/L	$150–400 \times 10^9$/L
Sodium	133 mmol/L	135–145 mmol/L
Potassium	3.3 mmol/L	3.5–5.0 mmol/L
Urea	6.1 mmol/L	2.5–6.7 mmmol/L
Creatinine	63 μmol/L	44–80 μmol/L
Amylase	75 IU/L	0–99 IU/L

An X-ray of the abdomen is performed and is shown in Fig. 1.1.

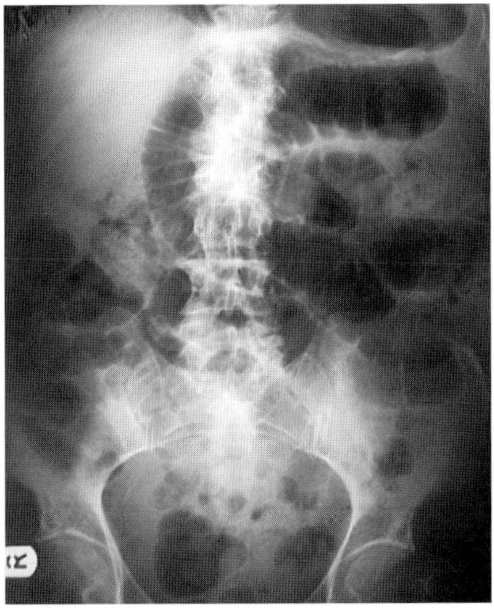

Figure 1.1 Plain X-ray of the abdomen.

Questions

- What is the cause of the X-ray appearances?
- What is the swelling?
- What are the anatomical boundaries?
- What is the initial treatment in this case?
- What is the differential diagnosis for a lump in the groin region?

ANSWER 1

This woman has a right-sided femoral hernia. The neck of the femoral hernia lies below and lateral to the pubic tubercle, differentiating it from an inguinal hernia which lies above and medial to the pubic tubercle. The X-ray shows small-bowel dilation as a result of obstruction due to trapped small bowel in the hernia sac. The high white cell count, temperature and tenderness may indicate strangulation of the hernia contents. The rigid borders of the femoral canal make strangulation more likely than in inguinal hernias.

! Relations of the femoral canal

- *Anteriorly*: inguinal ligament
- *Posteriorly*: superior ramus of the pubis and pectineus muscle
- *Medially*: body of pubis, pubic part of the inguinal ligament
- *Laterally*: femoral vein

The patient should be kept nil by mouth, and intravenous fluids and antibiotics begun. A nasogastric tube should be passed and blood taken for crossmatch. Theatres should then be informed and the patient taken for urgent surgery to reduce and repair the hernia, with careful inspection of the hernial sac contents. If the bowel is infarcted it will need to be resected.

! Differential diagnosis for a lump in the groin

- Inguinal hernia
- Femoral hernia
- Hydrocoele of the cord
- Hydrocoele of the canal of Nuck
- Lipoma of the cord
- Undescended testicle
- Ectopic testicle
- Saphena varix
- Iliofemoral aneurysm
- Lymph nodes
- Psoas abscess

KEY POINTS

- Femoral hernias are at high risk of strangulation.
- If strangulation is suspected urgent surgical correction is required.

CASE 2: RIGHT ILIAC FOSSA PAIN

History

A 19-year-old man presents with a 2-day history of abdominal pain. The pain started in the central abdomen and has now become constant and has shifted to the right iliac fossa. The patient has vomited twice today and is off his food. His motions were loose today, but there was no associated rectal bleeding.

Examination

The patient has a temperature of 37.8°C and a pulse rate of 110/min. On examination of his abdomen he has localized tenderness and guarding in the right iliac fossa. Urinalysis is clear.

INVESTIGATIONS

		Normal
Haemoglobin	14.2 g/dL	11.5–16.0 g/dL
Mean cell volume	86 fL	76–96 fL
White cell count	19×10^9/L	$4.0–11.0 \times 10^9$/L
Platelets	250×10^9/L	$150–400 \times 10^9$/L
Sodium	136 mmol/L	135–145 mmol/L
Potassium	3.5 mmol/L	3.5–5.0 mmol/L
Urea	5.0 mmol/L	2.5–6.7 mmmol/L
Creatinine	62 μmol/L	44–80 μmol/L
C-reactive protein	20 mg/L	<5 mg/L

Questions

- What is the likely diagnosis?
- What are the differential diagnoses for this condition?
- How would you manage this patient?
- What are the complications of any surgical intervention that may be required?

ANSWER 2

The history and the findings on examination strongly suggest acute appendicitis.

! The differential diagnoses of acute appendicitis

- mesenteric adenitis
- psoas abscess
- Meckel's diverticulum
- Crohn's disease
- non-specific abdominal pain

and additionally in females:

- ovarian cyst rupture
- ovarian torsion
- ectopic pregnancy (all females must have a pregnancy test)

The treatment is appendicectomy. The patient should be rehydrated with preoperative intravenous fluids, and receive analgesia. Antibiotics should be given if the diagnosis is clear and the decision for surgery has been made. Surgery should be carried out promptly in a patient who has signs of peritonitis, in order to avoid systemic toxicity. The appendix can be removed by open operation or laparoscopically.

! Complications

- Wound infection: reduced by using broad spectrum antibiotics
- Intra-abdominal collections and pelvic abscesses
- Prolonged ileus
- Fistulation between the appendix stump and the wound
- Deep vein thrombosis, pulmonary embolism, pneumonia, atelectasis
- Late complications: incisional hernia, adhesional obstruction

KEY POINT

- If the appendix is normal at the time of the operation, the small bowel should be inspected for the presence of a Meckel's diverticulum.

CASE 3: ABDOMINAL DISTENSION POST HIP REPLACEMENT

History

You are asked to review a 72-year-old man on the orthopaedic ward. He had a hemi-arthroplasty of his right hip 6 days earlier. He was recovering well initially but has now developed significant abdominal distension. He has not opened his bowels or passed flatus for the last 4 days. His previous medical history includes treatment for a transitional cell carcinoma of the bladder and an appendicectomy. He is also known to have a hiatus hernia. He gave up smoking 6 months ago.

Examination

His blood pressure is 114/88 mmHg and pulse rate is 98/min. The abdomen is significantly distended with mild generalized tenderness. The abdomen is resonant to percussion and a few bowel sounds are heard. There are no hernias, and digital rectal examination reveals an empty rectum.

INVESTIGATIONS

		Normal
Haemoglobin	10.2 g/dL	11.5–16.0 g/dL
White cell count	12.6×10^9/L	$4.0–11.0 \times 10^9$/L
Platelets	422×10^9/L	$150–400 \times 10^9$/L
Sodium	131 mmol/L	135–145 mmol/L
Potassium	3.2 mmol/L	3.5–5.0 mmol/L
Urea	5.7 mmol/L	2.5–6.7 mmmol/L
Creatinine	78 μmol/L	44–80 μmol/L

An X-ray of the abdomen is performed and is shown in Fig. 3.1.

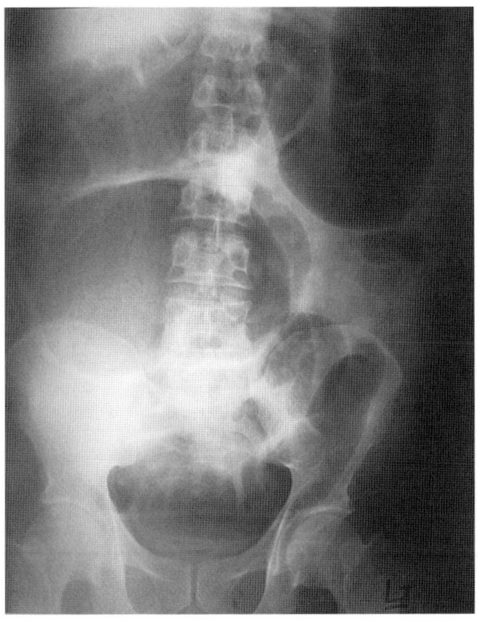

Figure 3.1 Plain X-ray of the abdomen.

Questions

- What is the diagnosis?
- Are there any patients at particular risk of developing this condition?
- What is the significance of the right iliac fossa pain in this setting?
- What does conservative treatment consist of?

ANSWER 3

The patient has large-bowel obstruction. When no mechanical cause is found for the obstruction the condition is referred to as a pseudo-obstruction. The pathogenesis of the condition is still unclear but abnormal colonic motility is thought to be a major factor. On the radiograph, air is seen throughout the colon down to the rectum making a mechanical cause unlikely. If this is unclear then a water-soluble contrast enema should be used to exclude a mechanical cause.

Pseudo-obstruction tends to occur in patients following trauma, severe infection or orthopaedic/cardiothoracic/pelvic surgery. Systemic causes include sepsis, metabolic abnormalities and drugs. The clinical features are marked abdominal distension, nausea, vomiting, absolute constipation, abdominal pain and high-pitched bowel sounds. The presence of a temperature with signs of peritonism suggests that the bowel is ischaemic and a perforation is imminent. This is most likely to occur in the caecum due to the distensibility of the bowel wall at this point. The patient should be examined carefully for tenderness in the right iliac fossa, and the caecal diameter noted on the radiograph. If the diameter increases to over 10 cm, then there is a significant risk of perforation.

Conservative treatment involves keeping the patient nil by mouth, intravenous fluids and nasogastric decompression. A flatus tube can be placed by rigid sigmoidoscopy to relieve some of the distension. Decompression is more effectively achieved by colonoscopy. Fluid and electrolyte abnormalities should be corrected and drugs affecting colonic motility discontinued, e.g. opiates.

KEY POINTS

- The overall mortality rate in pseudo-obstruction managed conservatively is approximately 15 per cent.
- This figure rises to 30 per cent in patients who require surgery and as high as 50–90 per cent with faecal peritonitis.

CASE 4: PERIANAL PAIN

History

A 28-year-old man presents to the emergency department complaining of anal and lower-back pain for the previous 36 h. He has tried taking simple analgesics with no benefit. The pain is progressively getting worse and he is now finding it uncomfortable to walk or sit down. He is otherwise fit and well and smokes 10 cigarettes a day.

Examination

Inspection of the anus reveals a 3 cm × 3 cm swelling at the anal margin. The swelling is warm, exquisitely tender and fluctuant. There is no other obvious abnormality.

Questions

- What is the diagnosis?
- What are the aetiological factors associated with this condition?
- How are these lesions anatomically classified?
- What treatment is required?

ANSWER 4

This patient has a perianal abscess. The organisms responsible tend to be either from the gut (*Bacteroides fragilis, E. coli* or enterococci) or from the skin (*Staphylococcus aureus*). Anorectal abscesses originate from infection arising in the cryptoglandular epithelium lining the anal canal. The internal anal sphincter can be breached through the crypts of Morgagni, which penetrate through the internal sphincter into the intersphincteric space. Once the infection passes into the intersphincteric space, it can spread easily into the adjacent perirectal spaces.

! Classification of anorectal abscesses

See Fig. 4.1.

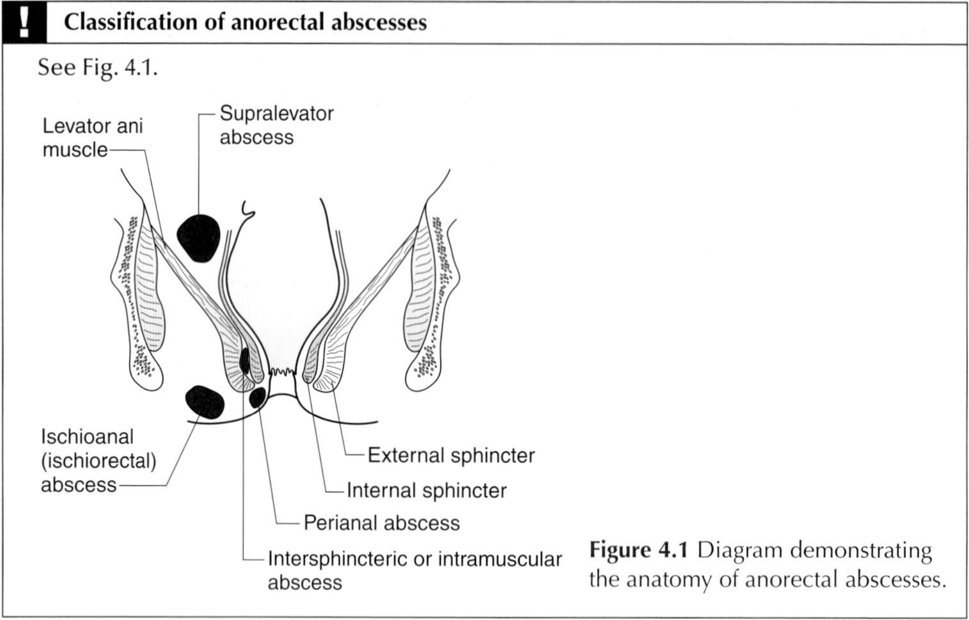

Figure 4.1 Diagram demonstrating the anatomy of anorectal abscesses.

! Aetiological factors for anorectal abscesses

- Idiopathic (vast majority)
- Crohn's disease
- Anorectal carcinoma
- Anal fissure
- Anal trauma/surgery
- Pelvic abscesses may arise secondary to inflammatory bowel disease or diverticulitis

The patient should have an examination under anaesthesia (EUA) with sigmoidoscopy to examine the bowel mucosa. The abscess should be treated by incision and drainage, and pus should be sent for culture. Skin organisms are less commonly associated with fistulae than gut organisms. Anorectal fistulas occur in 30–60 per cent of patients with anorectal abscesses. If a fistula is found at the time of incision and drainage, the location should be noted and the patient brought back once the sepsis has resolved.

KEY POINTS

- Anorectal fistulas occur in 30–60 per cent of patients with anorectal abscesses.
- Sigmoidoscopy and proctoscopy should be done at the time of surgery to examine for underlying pathology.

CASE 5: SUSPICIOUS MOLE

History

A 36-year-old Caucasian man presents to his general practitioner concerned that a mole has changed shape and increased in size over the preceding month. It is itchy but has not changed colour or bled. There is no relevant family history. He is fit and well otherwise. As part of his job he spends half the year in California. He smokes five cigarettes per day.

Examination

He appears well. Several moles are present over the neck and trunk. All appear benign, except the one he points out that he is concerned about. This is located on the left-hand side of his trunk and is black, measuring 1 × 1.5 cm. The lesion is non-tender with a slightly irregular surface. There is a surrounding pink halo around the lesion. The local lymph nodes are not enlarged. Abdominal, chest and neurological examination is normal.

Questions

- What is the most likely diagnosis?
- What treatment would you recommend?
- Why is it important to examine the abdomen and chest and assess neurology in such patients?
- What are the risk factors for this condition?
- What factors in the history of such patients would make you concerned?

ANSWER 5

The patient has malignant melanoma until proven otherwise. An excision biopsy should be recommended with a clear margin of 1–3 mm and full skin thickness. This is then assessed by a histopathologist. If malignant melanoma is confirmed, tumour thickness (Breslow score) and anatomical level of invasion (Clarke's stage) are ascertained. Both give important prognostic information. Treatment is predominantly surgical with wide local excision. Impalpable lesions should have a 1 cm clear margin and palpable lesions a 2 cm clear margin.

When examining patients with suspicious moles, lymphadenopathy must be sought, as this indicates spread of the malignant melanoma. In such cases, treatment will also include a lymph node dissection +/– radiotherapy, in addition to primary surgical excision. In cases with metastasis, malignant melanoma usually involves the lungs, liver and brain.

! Risk factors for malignant melanoma

- Sun exposure particularly intermittent
- Fair skin, blue eyes, red or blonde hair
- Dysplastic naevus syndrome
- Albinism
- Xeroderma pigmentosum
- Congenital giant hairy naevus
- Hutchinson's freckle
- Previous malignant melanoma
- Family history

! Factors in the history that are suggestive of malignant change in a mole

- Change in surface
- Itching
- Increase in size/shape/thickness
- Change in colour
- Bleeding/ulceration
- Brown/pink halo (spread into surrounding skin)/satellite nodules
- Enlarged local lymph nodes

KEY POINTS

- Patients should always be examined for associated lymphadenopathy.
- All specimens should be sent for urgent histological analysis.

CASE 6: ABDOMINAL PAIN, DISTENSION AND VOMITING

History

A 54-year-old man presents to the emergency department with a 4-day history of abdominal distension, central colicky abdominal pain, vomiting and constipation. On further questioning he says he has passed a small amount of flatus yesterday but none today. He has had a previous right-sided hemicolectomy 2 years ago for colonic carcinoma. He lives with his wife and has no known allergies.

Examination

His blood pressure and temperature are normal. The pulse is irregularly irregular at 90/min. He has obvious abdominal distension, but the abdomen is only mildly tender centrally. The hernial orifices are clear. There is no loin tenderness and the rectum is empty on digital examination. The bowel sounds are hyperactive and high pitched. Chest examination finds reduced air entry bibasally.

INVESTIGATIONS

		Normal
Haemoglobin	12.2 g/dL	11.5–16.0 g/dL
White cell count	10.6×10^9/L	$4.0–11.0 \times 10^9$/L
Platelets	435×10^9/L	$150–400 \times 10^9$/L
Sodium	136 mmol/L	135–145 mmol/L
Potassium	3.7 mmol/L	3.5–5.0 mmol/L
Urea	6.2 mmol/L	2.5–6.7 mmmol/L
Creatinine	77 μmol/L	44–80 μmol/L

An X-ray of the abdomen is performed and is shown in Fig. 6.1.

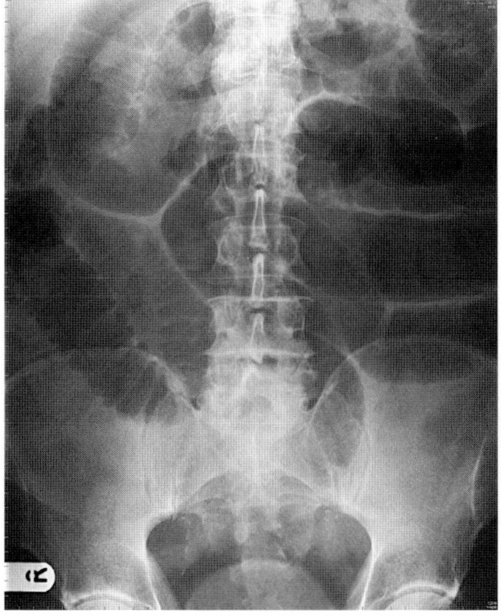

Figure 6.1 Plain X-ray of the abdomen.

Questions

- What is the diagnosis?
- What features on the X-ray point towards the diagnosis?
- How should the patient be managed initially?
- What are the common causes of this condition?

ANSWER 6

The diagnosis is small-bowel obstruction. In this case it is most likely to be secondary to adhesions from his previous abdominal surgery, but may also be due to recurrence of his cancer. Typical features on the X-ray include dilated gas-filled loops of bowel and air-fluid levels. Small bowel is distinguished from the large bowel by its valvular conniventes (radiologically transverse the whole diameter of the bowel). The large bowel has haustral folds, which do not fully transverse the diameter of the bowel. Small-bowel loops usually lie centrally and large-bowel loops lie peripherally. If a patient develops any systemic signs of sepsis or peritonism, then strangulation of the bowel should be considered. If this occurs, the patient will require urgent resuscitation and a laparotomy. If the patient is systemically well, with a diagnosis of adhesional obstruction, then management is as follows:

! Initial management

- Keep the patient nil by mouth
- In small-bowel obstruction there is substantial fluid loss and intravenous fluid resuscitation is necessary
- Regular observation
- Urinary catheter to monitor fluid balance
- Consider central venous line to monitor fluid balance in shocked patients
- Pass a nasogastric tube and perform regular aspirates
- Consider high-dependency unit (HDU)/intensive-care unit (ICU) transfer for optimization prior to surgery if required

! Aetiology of small-bowel obstruction

- Adhesions – common after previous abdominal/gynaecological surgery
- Incarcerated herniae, e.g. inguinal, femoral, paraumbilical, spigelian, incisional
- Gallstone ileus
- Inflammatory bowel disease
- Radiation enteritis
- Intussusception

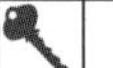

KEY POINT

- Early nasogastric tube decompression will relieve abdominal distension and prevent vomiting in small-bowel obstruction.

CASE 7: PER RECTAL BLEEDING

History

A 62-year-old Japanese businessman presents to the emergency department with significant bright red rectal bleeding for the last 6 h. He has no abdominal pain and has not vomited. There is no previous history of altered bowel habit. His appetite is normal and he reports no recent weight loss. Although he has lived in this country for 15 years, he has regular oesophagogastroduodenoscopy (OGD) because of a strong family history of stomach cancer. The last endoscopy was 2 months ago and was clear. He has recently been diagnosed with mild hypertension. He takes bendroflumethiazide 2.5 mg once daily and smokes 10 cigarettes per day.

Examination

He looks pale and sweaty. His blood pressure is 94/60 mmHg and his pulse is thready with a rate of 118/min. His temperature is normal. His abdomen is soft with no evidence of distension. The rest of his examination is unremarkable. Rectal examination reveals altered blood mixed with the stool and there are some blood clots on the glove. Rigid sigmoidoscopy was unsuccessful due to the presence of blood and faeces.

INVESTIGATIONS

		Normal
Haemoglobin	7.4 g/dL	11.5–16.0 g/dL
WCC	13.6×10^9/L	$4.0–11.0 \times 10^9$/L
Platelets	404×10^9/L	$150–400 \times 10^9$/L
Sodium	134 mmol/L	135–145 mmol/L
Potassium	4.8 mmol/L	3.5–5.0 mmol/L
Urea	8.6 mmol/L	2.5–6.7 mmmol/L
Creatinine	115 μmol/L	44–80 μmol/L
International normalized ratio (INR)	1.2 IU	1 IU

Questions

- What is the immediate management?
- What is the differential diagnosis?
- If the bleeding does not settle what other investigations may be necessary?
- What are the indications for surgical treatment?

ANSWER 7

The immediate management is to obtain intravenous access with two large-bore cannulae in the anterior cubital fossae. Bloods should be taken for a full blood count, coagulation screen, renal function and a crossmatch for at least four units. Intravenous fluids should be started and a urinary catheter inserted to monitor hourly urine output. The patient is best monitored closely until he becomes stable with regular observations. Central venous monitoring should be considered and transfer to a high-dependency unit may be necessary.

! Differential diagnoses

- Diverticular disease
- Inflammatory bowel disease
- Angiodysplasia
- Infective colitis, e.g. *Campylobacter, Salmonella, E. Coli, Clostridium* species
- Ischaemic colitis, e.g. mesenteric infarction/embolism
- Radiation colitis
- Haemorrhoids
- Neoplasia
- Meckel's diverticulum

Often the bleeding settles with conservative management. If the bleeding continues, an OGD should be done first to rule out an upper gastrointestinal cause for the bleeding. Colonoscopy can then be performed to assess the large bowel for a cause. Unfortunately, because of the presence of blood, views are often poor. If the approximate area of affected bowel can be established, it allows better planning for surgical intervention.

If the bleeding is quite dramatic, mesenteric angiography should be considered, to delineate the anatomy and identify any bleeding vessels. Selective embolization may be employed to stop the bleeding in certain cases. With this technique, sites of bleeding can only be located if the blood loss is over 1 mL/min. If the source of bleeding is not known and other measures have failed, the patient may require a sub-total colectomy.

KEY POINT

- Haemoglobin should be repeated at 12 h as anaemia may not be evident on the initial sample.

CASE 8: SWELLING IN THE GROIN

History

A 38-year-old computer engineer is referred to surgical outpatients complaining of pain in the right groin. He has noticed this over the last few months and his pain is worse on exertion. He has also noticed an intermittent swelling. He is otherwise fit and well. There is a family history of bowel cancer. He is a smoker of 25 cigarettes per day and drinks 10 units of alcohol per week.

Examination

He is apyrexial with normal blood pressure and pulse. The abdomen is grossly normal but there is some tenderness in the right groin. The patient is asked to stand. In the right groin, there is a swelling which is more pronounced when the patient coughs. The other groin and the scrotal examination are normal.

Questions

- What is the likely diagnosis?
- What are the anatomical boundaries?
- What are the complications associated with this condition?
- How should the patient be treated?

ANSWER 8

The patient is likely to have an inguinal hernia. The boundaries of the inguinal canal are:

- *anteriorly*: the external oblique and internal oblique muscle in the lateral third
- *posteriorly*: the transversalis fascia and the conjoint tendon (merging of the pubic attachments of the internal oblique and transverse abdominal aponeurosis into a common tendon)
- *roof*: arching fibres of the internal oblique and transverse abdominus muscles
- *floor*: the inguinal ligament.

Inguinal herniae are more common in males and in the right groin. Indirect inguinal hernial sacs are found lateral to the inferior epigastric vessels at the deep inguinal ring. Direct hernias are found medial to the inferior epigastric vessels and are a result of a weakness in the posterior wall. This distinction between the two can only be made with certainty at the time of surgery. The key in distinguishing between femoral and inguinal herniae is their point of reduction. Femoral herniae reduce below and lateral to the pubic tubercle, and inguinal herniae above and medial to the tubercle.

! Complications of an inguinal hernia

- Incarceration, i.e. irreducible
- Bowel obstruction
- Strangulation
- Reduction-en-masse: reduction through the abdominal wall without pushing bowel contents out of the hernial sac

The patient should have a surgical repair of the hernia. This can be done by either an open or laparoscopic approach. Both involve reduction of the hernia and placement of a mesh to prevent recurrence.

KEY POINTS

- Indirect and symptomatic direct hernias should be repaired to prevent the risk of future strangulation.
- Irreducible inguinal hernias should be repaired promptly to avoid strangulation.
- Easily reducible symptomless direct hernias, need not always be repaired, especially in elderly patients with significant comorbidities.

CASE 9: DIFFERENTIAL DIAGNOSIS OF LOWER ABDOMINAL PAIN

History

A 22-year-old woman presents to the emergency department complaining of lower abdominal pain. This has steadily increased in severity over the previous 24 h and woke her from her sleep. The pain is constant, and simple analgesia has not helped. She has vomited once in the department. Her menses are regular and she is now on day 12 of her cycle. There is no history of vaginal discharge or urinary symptoms. She has no children. She has not undergone any previous surgery but has a history of sexually transmitted disease 2 years ago, treated with antibiotics. There is no other relevant medical history. She takes no current medication and has no allergies. She is a non-smoker.

Examination

Her blood pressure is 110/72 mmHg and pulse rate is 110/min. Her temperature is 38.2°C and there is lower abdominal tenderness, more marked in the right iliac fossa, with some rebound tenderness. There are no palpable masses and the loins are not tender. Digital rectal examination is normal. Bimanual per vaginal examination reveals adnexal tenderness on the right.

INVESTIGATIONS

		Normal
Haemoglobin	14.7 g/dL	11.5–16.0 g/dL
White cell count	16.6×10^9/L	$4.0–11.0 \times 10^9$/L
Platelets	367×10^9/L	$150–400 \times 10^9$/L
Sodium	139 mmol/L	135–145 mmol/L
Potassium	4.1 mmol/L	3.5–5.0 mmol/L
Urea	5.6 mmol/L	2.5–6.7 mmmol/L
Creatinine	74 μmol/L	44–80 μmol/L
C-reactive protein (CRP)	145 mg/L	<5 mg/L

Urine dipstick: NAD (nothing abnormal detected)

Urinary β human chorionic gonadotrophin (HCG): negative

Questions

- What is the differential diagnosis?
- How should the patient be managed initially?
- If you are unsure of the diagnosis, how should you proceed?

ANSWER 9

The two main differential diagnoses are pelvic inflammatory disease and acute appendicitis. The young female with right iliac fossa pain is often difficult to diagnose. The other differential diagnoses of right iliac fossa pain mimicking appendicitis are shown below.

! Differential diagnoses

- *Gynaecological*
  - pelvic inflammatory disease (salpingitis, salpingo-oophoritis, tubo-ovarian abscess, endometritis, Fitz-Hugh–Curtis syndrome)
  - ruptured ovarian cyst
  - ovarian torsion
  - haemorrhage/rupture of ovarian mass
- *Surgical*
  - Crohn's disease
  - mesenteric adenitis
  - gastroenteritis
  - diverticulitis (caecal or left sided with a floppy sigmoid lying centrally or on the right of the midline)
  - Meckel's diverticulitis
  - acute cholecystitis
- *Urological*
  - acute pyelonephritis
  - ureteric colic

The high white cell count, raised CRP and tenderness in the right iliac fossa make appendicitis the most likely diagnosis in this patient. In clear-cut cases of appendicitis the patient is taken to theatre for appendicectomy. If the diagnosis is most likely gynaecological, the patient should be referred to the gynaecologists for a transvaginal ultrasound scan and high vaginal swabs. Where there is doubt, the patient can be taken for diagnostic laparoscopy. If the appendix is abnormal it can then be removed laparoscopically.

KEY POINT

- A full gynaecological history should be taken in female patients.

CASE 10: SMALL-BOWEL ANOMALY

History

A 14-year-old boy presented to the emergency department with a 24 h history of increasing abdominal pain. The pain localized to the right iliac fossa and a diagnosis of acute appendicitis was made. At operation the appendix was found to be normal and the anomaly shown in Fig. 10.1 was found in a loop of small bowel.

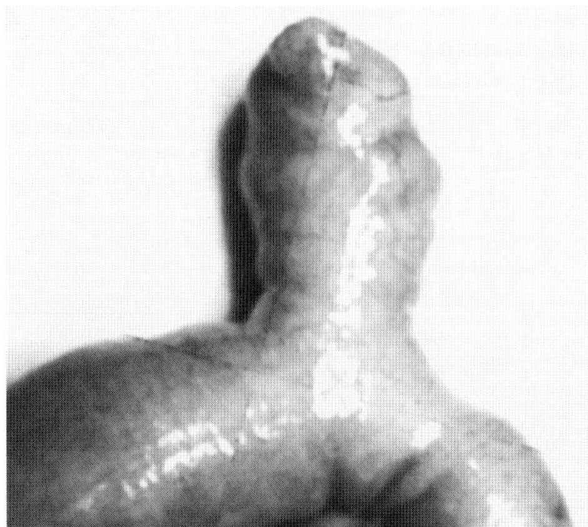

Figure 10.1 Operative picture of the small bowel.

Questions

- What is the diagnosis?
- What are the characteristics of this anomaly?
- How can this present?
- How would you deal with this intra-operative finding?

ANSWER 10

The photograph demonstrates a Meckel's diverticulum located on the anti-mesenteric border of a segment of ileum. This is a remnant of the omphalomesenteric duct. The 'rule of twos' is associated with this condition, i.e. it is present in 2 per cent of the population, it is 2 inches long and located 2 feet from the ileocaecal valve. A Meckel's diverticulum may be lined by small-intestinal, colonic or gastric mucosa, and it may contain aberrant pancreatic tissue.

The mode of presentation may be:

- inflammation and perforation of the diverticulum presenting with abdominal pain and peritonitis, mimicking acute appendicitis
- rectal bleeding from peptic ulceration caused by acid secretion from the ectopic gastric mucosa
- intestinal obstruction from intussusception or entrapment of the bowel in a mesodiverticular band or a fibrous band that may connect the apex of the diverticulum to the umbilicus or anterior abdominal wall.

Tumours may also develop inside a Meckel's diverticulum.

The diverticulum should be removed by a segmental small-bowel resection. A symptomless diverticulum that is an incidental finding at laparotomy should not be excised, but the patient should be informed of its existence.

KEY POINT

- Patients should be made aware if an asymptomatic Meckel's diverticulum is found at the time of surgery.

CASE 11: A RECTAL MASS

History

A 70-year-old man was seen in the surgical outpatient clinic complaining of a 3-month history of loose stools. He normally opens his bowels once a day, but has recently been passing loose motions up to four times a day. The motions have been associated with the passage of blood clots and fresh blood mixed within the stools. His appetite has been normal, but he reports a 2-stone weight loss. The past history was otherwise unremarkable. His father died from cancer at the age of 45 years, but he is unsure of the origin.

Examination

No pallor or lymphadenopathy is present. The abdomen is soft and non-tender with no palpable masses. Digital rectal examination is normal.

INVESTIGATIONS

Rigid sigmoidoscopy reveals a mass located approximately 11 cm from the anal verge (Fig. 11.1).

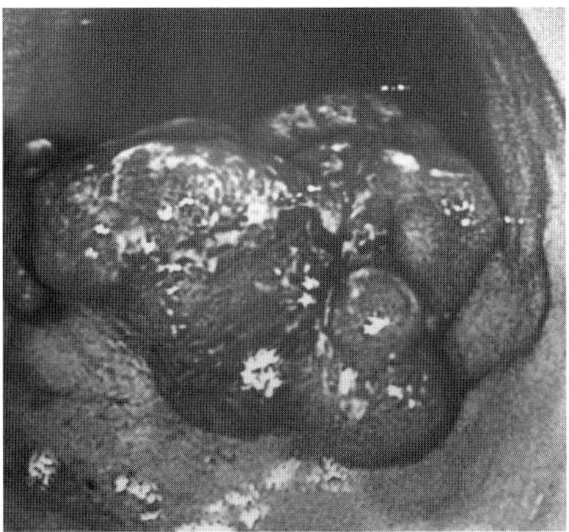

Figure 11.1 Lesion on sigmoidoscopy.

Questions

- What is the likely diagnosis?
- How should the patient be investigated?
- What are the options for treatment?
- Which are the worrying symptoms in the patient's history?

ANSWER 11

A sessile mass is seen occupying approximately half of the bowel wall circumference. A biopsy of the lesion should be taken at the time of sigmoidoscopy to confirm the diagnosis of rectal cancer.

Blood tests including full blood count, liver function tests and tumour markers (e.g. carcinoembryonic antigen [CEA]) should be arranged. An urgent colonoscopy is required to determine whether there are any synchronous cancers (5 per cent) or synchronus polyps (75 per cent) in the rest of the large bowel.

The patient should be staged using computerized tomography (CT) of the chest and abdomen to check for chest, mediastinal and intra-abdominal metastases. Magnetic resonance imaging (MRI) of the pelvis is used to ascertain the depth of tumour invasion through the rectal wall and any regional nodal metastases. For tumours located above approximately 5 cm from the anal verge, an anterior resection is carried out with or without a temporary defunctioning colostomy. If the tumour is less than 5 cm from the anal verge, then abdomino-perineal resection of the anus and rectum maybe required with a permanent end colostomy.

For tumours penetrating the rectal wall preoperative radiotherapy is beneficial, and more recently a combination of chemotherapy and radiotherapy has been advocated for some tumours.

KEY POINTS

The following symptoms should prompt urgent colorectal assessment:

- rectal bleeding with a change in bowel habit to looser stools and/or frequency of defaecation persistent for 6 weeks
- patients aged over 60 years with a change in bowel habit as above without rectal bleeding and persistent for 6 weeks
- patients aged over 60 years with rectal bleeding persistently without anal symptoms
- a definite palpable right-sided abdominal mass
- a definite palpable rectal mass (not pelvic)
- iron-deficiency anaemia without an obvious cause below 10 g/dL in postmenopausal women and below 11 g/dL in all men.

CASE 12: INVESTIGATION OF ANAEMIA

History

A 68-year-old man is referred by his general practitioner (GP) with a 6-week history of lethargy and breathlessness on walking. He is off his food and has lost 2 stone in weight over the previous 2 months. He reports no rectal bleeding or change in bowel habit. His father died at the age of 58 years from a colonic tumour. He is otherwise well and not on any regular medication. His GP referred him to the colorectal clinic, as he was concerned about his blood results and his strong family history of colorectal cancer. An oesophagogastroduodenoscopy (OGD) had been previously requested by the GP and was normal.

Examination

On examination, his conjunctivae are pale and he looks cachectic. There is no jaundice or palpable lymphadenopathy. The chest is clear and the heart sounds are normal. Examination of the abdomen reveals a fullness in the right iliac fossa. There is no associated hepatomegaly. Digital rectal examination and sigmoidoscopy to 18 cm are normal.

INVESTIGATIONS

		Normal
Haemoglobin	7.4 g/dL	11.5–16.0 g/dL
Mean cell volume	70 fL	76–96 fL
White cell count	6×10^9/L	$4.0–11.0 \times 10^9$/L
Platelets	250×10^9/L	$150–400 \times 10^9$/L
Sodium	132 mmol/L	135–145 mmol/L
Potassium	3.8 mmol/L	3.5–5.0 mmol/L
Urea	16 mmol/L	2.5–6.7 mmmol/L
Creatinine	6.2 μmol/L	44–80 μmol/L

A computerized tomography (CT) of the abdomen and pelvis (Fig. 12.1) and a colonoscopy are organized.

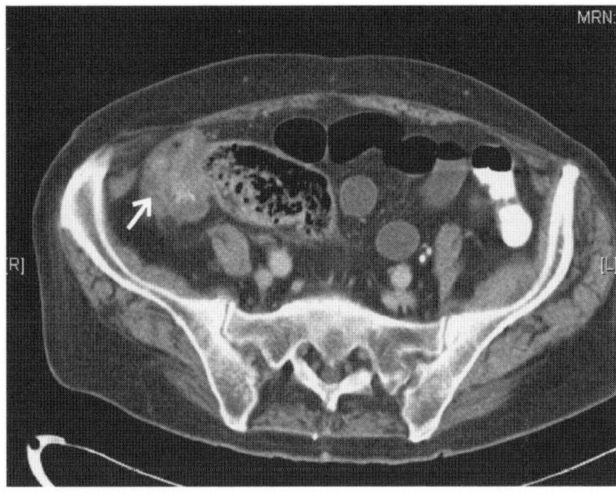

Figure 12.1 Computerized tomography of the abdomen.

Questions

- How should microcytic anaemia be investigated?
- What is the most likely diagnosis in this case?
- What further investigations are required for this patient?
- What treatment is appropriate?

ANSWER 12

Iron-deficiency anaemia should be firstly confirmed by a low serum ferritin, red cell microcytosis or hypochromia. The patient should then have their urine checked for haematuria, a rectal examination, and should be screened for coeliac disease. OGD and colonoscopy should be performed to exclude malignancy. One of the most common causes of iron-deficiency anaemia is from medications such as aspirin or other non-steroidal anti-inflammatory drugs.

The CT scan in this patient shows a caecal tumour. These can present insidiously and may only present with iron-deficiency anaemia. Further investigations should include liver function tests and a carcinoembryonic antigen (CEA) tumour marker level. A CT scan of the chest, abdomen and pelvis will delineate the nature of the mass and any metastatic disease. A colonoscopy provides a tissue diagnosis and will rule out any metachronous tumours in the large bowel.

In the absence of metastatic disease, the patient should undergo right hemicolectomy. Adjuvant chemotherapy may be required, depending on the depth of the resected tumour and involvement of the local lymph nodes. If metastatic disease is present then a palliative resection should be considered in patients with anaemia or obstruction.

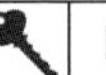

KEY POINT

- Serum ferritin should be checked in patients with microcytic anaemia.

CASE 13: ABDOMINAL DISTENSION AND PAIN

History

A 70-year-old man has been sent to the emergency department from a nursing home, complaining of intermittent sharp abdominal pain. He has not opened his bowels for 5 days. He suffered a major stroke in the past and requires constant nursing care. He has a history of chronic constipation. Previous medical history includes chronic obstructive airways disease for which he is on regular inhalers. He is allergic to penicillin and is an ex-smoker.

Examination

His blood pressure is 110/74 mmHg and the pulse rate is 112/min. His temperature is 37.8°C. There is gross abdominal distension with tenderness, most marked on the left-hand side. The abdomen is resonant to percussion and digital rectal examination reveals an empty rectum. There is a soft systolic murmur and mild scattered inspiratory wheeze on auscultation of the chest.

INVESTIGATIONS

An X-ray of the abdomen is performed and is shown in Fig. 13.1.

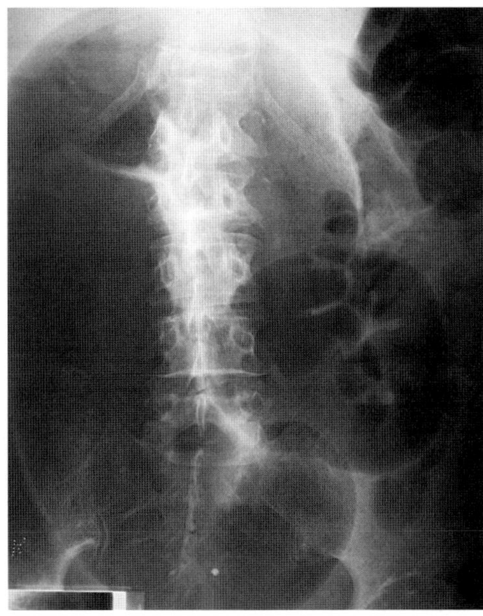

Figure 13.1 Plain X-ray of the abdomen.

Questions

- What does the abdominal X-ray show?
- What other radiological investigation could be employed if the diagnosis was in doubt?
- How should the patient be managed?
- What is the explanation for the pathology?

ANSWER 13

The X-ray shows a sigmoid volvulus. The sigmoid colon is grossly dilated and has an inverted U-tube shape. The involved bowel wall is usually oedematous and can form a dense central white line on the radiograph. On either side, the dilated loops of apposed bowel give the characteristic 'coffee bean' sign. X-ray appearances are diagnostic in 70 per cent of patients.

If there is doubt about the diagnosis, a water-soluble contrast may be helpful in showing a classical 'bird's beak' appearance representing the tapered lumen of the colon.

! Treatment of sigmoid volvulus

- Keep patient nil by mouth
- Intravenous access and fluids
- Fluid balance monitoring
- Routine bloods and crossmatch
- Erect chest X-ray/abdominal X-ray
- Decompression with rigid sigmoidoscopy and insertion of a flatus tube once the diagnosis is confirmed on abdominal X-ray

The flatus tube is left *in situ* for approximately 48 h and is often only a temporary measure. Colonoscopy can be used to decompress the bowel and may resolve the volvulus. Urgent laparotomy will be required if decompression is not possible or in cases of suspected gangrene/perforation (fever, leucocytosis, peritonism, free air under the diaphragm on erect chest radiography). The patient's fitness for surgery, prognosis and quality of life should be considered before proceeding to laparotomy. It may be appropriate to use only conservative treatments in some patients.

Sigmoid volvulus is predisposed to by a long, narrow mesocolon, chronic constipation or a high-roughage diet. The rotation of the gut can lead to obstruction and intestinal ischaemia. The sigmoid is the commonest part of the colon for this to occur, although the caecum and splenic flexure are other potential sites.

KEY POINT

- In the presence of peritonitis or pneumoperitoneum, the patient should be considered for urgent laparotomy.

CASE 14: ANAL PAIN

History

A 32-year-old man presents to the colorectal outpatient clinic with an 8-week history of pain on defaecation. The pain is around the anus and typically lasts an hour after passing stool. He normally suffers with constipation but this has now worsened as he is reluctant to pass motion because of the pain. He intermittently notices a small amount of fresh blood on the tissue paper after wiping himself. He has no family history of inflammatory bowel disease or colorectal cancer. He is otherwise well and takes no regular medications.

Examination

The patient appears well with no evidence of pallor, jaundice or lymphadenopathy. Abdominal examination is unremarkable. Examination of the anus reveals a small linear defect in the skin at the 6 o'clock position. Rectal examination could not be performed as it caused too much discomfort for the patient.

Questions

- What is the most likely diagnosis?
- What are the typical findings on examination?
- What are the differential diagnoses?
- What treatment would you recommend?

ANSWER 14

The most likely diagnosis is an anal fissure – this refers to a longitudinal tear in the anoderm within the distal one-third of the anal canal. Examination typically reveals a linear tear in the midline and posteriorly. Anterior fissures are more common in female patients. Chronic fissures are associated with skin tags, and the exposed fibres of the internal sphincter may be visible at their base. Anal fissures are common in patients with Crohn's disease and ulcerative colitis.

! Differential diagnoses

- Perianal haematoma
- Anorectal abscess
- Anorectal carcinoma
- Anal warts
- Anal herpes

More than half of acute fissures will heal with conservative treatment. This should include the use of laxatives, high dietary fibre, fruit and plenty of fluids to ensure the stool is soft. Topical local anaesthetic (e.g. lidocaine) can be used for pain relief. Non-healing fissures may respond to the use of topical 0.2 per cent glyceryltrinitrate ointment. This ointment can cause headaches and dizziness, so is not suitable for all patients. Some centres now advocate the direct injection of botulinum toxin into the anal sphincter to relieve spasm and promote healing. Lateral sphincterotomy has been shown to heal the vast majority of fissures within a few weeks but is associated with a small risk of incontinence and requires a general anaesthetic.

KEY POINT

- Laxatives, high dietary fibre, fruit and plenty of fluids are effective conservative treatments for anal fissures.

CASE 15: ABSOLUTE CONSTIPATION

History

A 70-year-old man presents with a 4-day history of colicky lower abdominal pain. He has been vomiting for the past 2 days and last opened his bowels 3 days ago. He has been unable to pass flatus for the past 24 h. He reports a 2-stone weight loss in the past year but is otherwise fit with no other past medical history of note. He currently lives on his own and leads an active life, walking his dog every day.

Examination

He is afebrile with a pulse rate of 100/min and a blood pressure of 100/50 mmHg. Cardiovascular and respiratory examinations are unremarkable. The abdomen is distended and tympanic to percussion with lower abdominal tenderness. The bowel sounds are 'tinkling'. The hernial orifices are empty and digital rectal examination reveals an empty rectum.

INVESTIGATIONS

An X-ray of the abdomen is performed and is shown in Fig. 15.1.

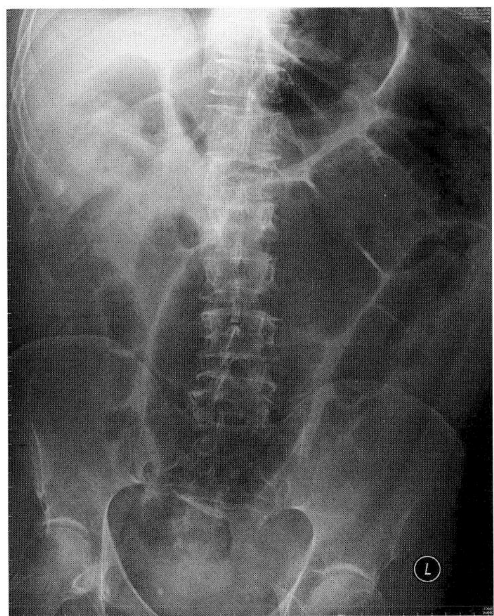

Figure 15.1 Plain X-ray of the abdomen.

Questions

- What is the likely diagnosis?
- What are the possible causes?
- Which further investigations are required?

ANSWER 15

The X-ray demonstrates large-bowel obstruction. Large-bowel obstruction classically presents with lower abdominal pain, abdominal distension and absolute constipation. Vomiting is a late feature. The common causes of large-bowel obstruction are listed below:

- *carcinoma*: approximately 15 per cent of colorectal cancers present with obstruction and roughly 25 per cent are found to have distant metastases at the time of presentation
- *diverticulitis*: repeated episodes of diverticulitis can lead to fibrosis and narrowing of the colonic lumen
- *volvulus*: sigmoid volvulus typically occurs in older individuals with a history of constipation and straining. Caecal volvulus is seen in younger patients and is associated with a congenital defect in the peritoneum, resulting in inadequate fixation of the caecum
- *intussusception*: intussusception is most commonly seen in children. Approximately 70 per cent of adult intussusceptions are caused by tumours
- *colonic pseudo-obstruction*: pseudo-obstruction or Ogilvie syndrome is seen most often in the elderly patient with chronic or severe illness.

In approximately 20 per cent of patients, the ileocaecal valve is competent resulting in a 'closed-loop' obstruction which does not allow decompression into the small bowel. The large bowel gradually dilates with maximal dilatation occurring in the caecum. Gross dilation (>10 cm) with tenderness over the caecum is a sign of impending perforation and requires prompt surgery. Decompression of the large bowel with a loop colostomy is the safest procedure to perform in the first instance. Some centres are now using colonic stents to relieve obstruction, but these are not available at all institutions. More definitive surgery can then be planned after optimization and further imaging.

A contrast enema can be used to determine the level of the obstruction and if it is complete. If the patient is stable and is suspected of having a tumour, then a staging computerized tomography should be done.

The barium enema demonstrates a stenosis at the rectosigmoid junction secondary to a tumour (arrow in Fig. 15.2).

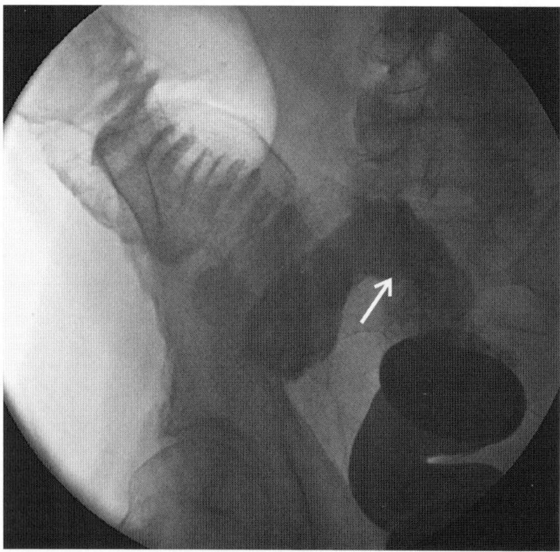

Figure 15.2 Barium enema demonstrating a stricture at the rectosigmoid junction (arrow).

KEY POINTS

Causes of large-bowel obstruction are:

- carcinoma
- diverticulitis
- volvulus
- intussusception
- colonic pseudo-obstruction.

CASE 16: LEFT ILIAC FOSSA PAIN

History

You are called to see a 66-year-old woman in the emergency department, who is complaining of a 5-day history of increasing left iliac fossa pain. She vomited once yesterday and has opened her bowels normally today. She usually suffers with constipation. The pain is severe and constant with no relieving factors. She has had one previous episode a year ago, which was treated with antibiotics. She was investigated once her symptoms had subsided, but is unclear about the final diagnosis.

Examination

She looks flushed, with dry mucous membranes and is febrile at 37.9°C. The pulse is 100/min with a blood pressure of 110/70 mmHg. Abdominal examination reveals localized tenderness and peritonism in the left iliac fossa. The rectum contains soft faeces on digital rectal examination. The previous investigation from a year ago is shown in Fig. 16.1.

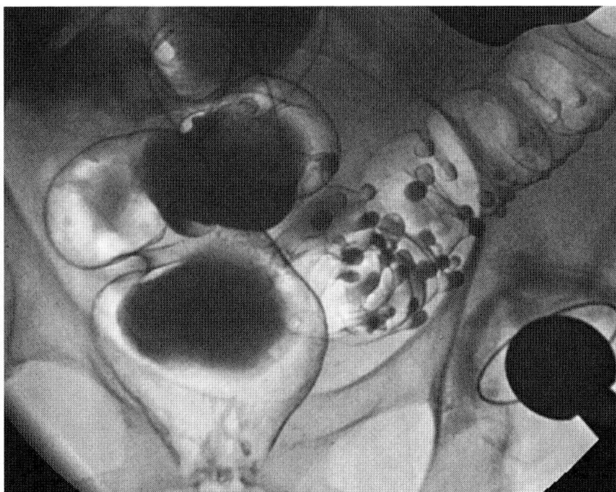

Figure 16.1 Previous investigation.

Questions

- What is the above investigation and what does it show?
- What is the likely diagnosis?
- What treatment would you initiate?
- What are the possible complications?
- How can the patient prevent further episodes?

ANSWER 16

The study shown is a barium enema. There are multiple diverticula of the sigmoid colon giving a diagnosis of diverticular disease. Diverticula are outpouchings of the mucous membrane alongside the taenia coli, at the entry point of the supplying blood vessels. Diverticular disease is very common, with over 60 per cent of the population affected by the age of 80 years. It is more common in developed countries due to low-fibre diets. The low-bulk stool leads to increased segmentation of the colon during propulsion, causing increased intraluminal pressure and formation of diverticula. They are found most commonly in the sigmoid colon (95–98 per cent of diverticula), but any part of the bowel may be affected.

The majority of patients with diverticula remain symptomless. Fifteen per cent complain of colicky abdominal pain without inflammation (diverticulosis), and 5 per cent develop acute diverticulitis. The impaction of faecal material in the neck of the diverticulum leads to trapping of bacteria. The bacteria then replicate in the occluded lumen leading to infection and inflammation. Diverticular disease is also a common cause of lower gastrointestinal bleeding. The small blood vessels, which are stretched over the dome of the diverticula, can rupture causing bleeding.

Initial investigations should include urinalysis, blood tests, blood cultures and a plain abdominal X-ray. Treatment should commence with intravenous access, intravenous fluids, analgesia, oxygen, broad-spectrum antibiotics and thromboprophylaxis. The patient should be monitored closely. Patients who do not improve after 24–48 h of treatment with antibiotics require further investigation with a computerized tomography (CT) scan of the abdomen to exclude a diverticular abscess. Patients in whom a diverticular perforation is suspected may require a laparotomy. Barium enema will confirm the diagnosis of diverticular disease, but this should not be performed in the acute setting. Once an acute episode has resolved, the patient should be commenced on a high-roughage diet to reduce the incidence of further attacks.

! Complications of diverticular disease

- Diverticulitis
- Pericolic abscess
- Colonic stricture
- Fistulation: vagina, bladder, skin
- Bacterial peritonitis: secondary to rupture of a pericolic abscess
- Faecal peritonitis: due to perforation of a diverticulum

KEY POINTS

- Over 60 per cent of the population have diverticular disease by the age of 80 years.
- The majority of cases of diverticulitis will settle with conservative management.

CASE 17: BRIGHT RED RECTAL BLEEDING

History

A 43-year-old man attends the surgical outpatient clinic complaining of intermittent bleeding per rectum for the past 2 months. The blood is always bright red, separate from the stool and drips into the pan. He also complains of itching around the anus. There is no other past medical history of note.

Examination

Abdominal examination is unremarkable. Rectal examination and proctoscopy shows internal haemorrhoids at the 3 and 7 o'clock positions.

Questions

- What are the differential diagnoses?
- What other examinations are required?
- How would you classify haemorrhoids?
- What are the treatments for haemorrhoids?

ANSWER 17

The most likely cause for the per rectal bleeding is haemorrhoids. Haemorrhoids are congested vascular cushions containing dilated veins and small arteries. They arise from the connective tissue in the anal canal and are classically described as lying in the 3, 7 and 11 o'clock positions. A low-fibre diet results in straining with defecation, causing engorgement of the tissue. This leads to enlargement of the cushions and prolapse. Pregnancy and abnormally high tension of the internal sphincter muscle can also cause haemorrhoidal problems.

! Differential diagnoses

- Anal fissure
- Perianal haematoma
- Carcinoma
- Anal polyp
- Inflammatory bowel disease

Sigmoidoscopy is mandatory to exclude rectal pathology up to the rectosigmoid junction. If there is any doubt as to the cause of bleeding, especially in the older patient, a flexible sigmoidoscopy or full colonoscopy should be carried out.

Haemorrhoids can be classified as:

- *first-degree haemorrhoids*: remain in the rectum
- *second-degree haemorrhoids*: prolapse through the anus on defecation but reduce spontaneously
- *third-degree haemorrhoids*: prolapse but require manual reduction
- *fourth-degree haemorrhoids*: prolapse and cannot be reduced.

Patients should be advised to take plenty of fluid, fruit, fibre and laxatives to keep the stool soft and to avoid straining. Treatments include phenol injections into the submucosa above the haemorrhoid and/or rubber-band ligation. Large second-degree and third-degree piles may require haemorrhoidectomy.

KEY POINT

- Eighty per cent of patients will not require surgical intervention.

CASE 18: CHANGE IN BOWEL HABIT

History

You are asked to see a 69-year-old retired baker in the outpatient clinic. For the past 7 weeks he has been passing more frequent stools (3–4 times per day). The motions are looser than normal, but do not contain any blood. He has lost a stone in weight in the past 6 months. Past history includes a fractured femur 8 years ago and an appendicectomy at the age of 20 years. His mother had ulcerative colitis. He is very active and a keen golfer.

Examination

The temperature is 36.5°C, the pulse rate is 69/min and the blood pressure is 150/85 mmHg. The abdomen is soft and non-tender with no masses or organomegaly. Digital rectal examination is unremarkable and rigid sigmoidoscopy to 20 cm does not show any abnormality.

Urgent investigation is requested and shown below.

INVESTIGATIONS

		Normal
Haemoglobin	14.2 g/dL	11.5–16.0 g/dL
Mean cell volume	86 fL	76–96 fL
White cell count	4.1×10^9/L	$4.0–11.0 \times 10^9$/L
Platelets	220×10^9/L	$150–400 \times 10^9$/L
Sodium	141 mmol/L	135–145 mmol/L
Potassium	4.6 mmol/L	3.5–5.0 mmol/L
Urea	7.1 mmol/L	2.5–6.7 mmmol/L
Creatinine	53 μmol/L	44–80 μmol/L
C-reactive protein	1 mg/L	<5 mg/L
Carcinoembryonic antigen	550 ng/mL	<2.5 ng/mL

A barium enema is performed (Fig. 18.1).

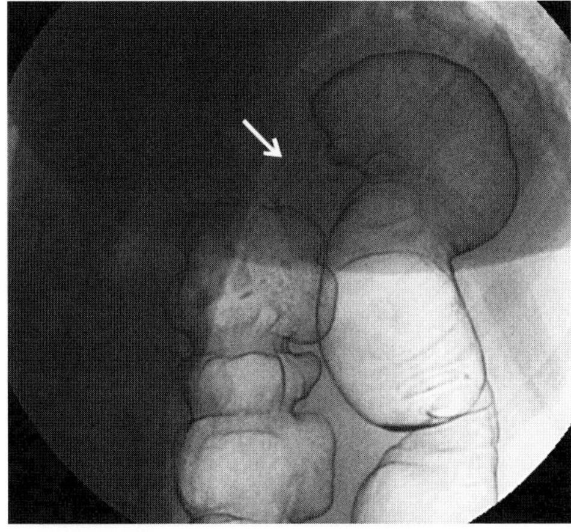

Figure 18.1 Barium enema.

Questions

- What does the barium enema in Fig. 18.1 show?
- What investigation is required for adequate preoperative staging?
- How can the tumour be staged upon histological examination of the resected specimen?
- Which groups of patients are at risk of developing colorectal cancer?

ANSWER 18

The study shown is a barium enema in a patient with a tumour at the splenic flexure (arrow). The appearance is typical of the narrowing of the colon lumen caused by an 'apple-core lesion'.

A colonoscopy would help to delineate the pathology within the colon and would allow biopsy to provide a tissue diagnosis. The colon can also be examined for synchronous tumours (found in 3 per cent). A computerized tomography (CT) scan of the chest, abdomen and pelvis is then required to stage the tumour and to determine operability. Once resected the tumour is staged by the Dukes' classification.

! Dukes' staging for pathological staging of colorectal cancer

- *A*: carcinoma not breaching the muscularis propria
- *B*: carcinoma breaching the muscularis propria but no involvement of local lymph nodes
- *C*: carcinoma involving local lymph nodes
- *D*: carcinoma with distant metastases
- *Five year survival*: 90 per cent, 70 per cent and 30 per cent for Stages A, B and C respectively.

Colorectal cancer is the second commonest cancer causing death in the UK, with over 19 000 new cases diagnosed each year. Most cancers are thought to arise within pre-existing adenomas. Right-sided lesions can present with iron-deficiency anaemia, weight loss or a right iliac fossa mass. Left-sided lesions present with alteration in bowel habit, rectal bleeding, or as an emergency with obstruction or perforation. Adjuvant radiotherapy is given for rectal cancer either pre- or postoperatively to prevent local recurrence. Adjuvant chemotherapy improves survival in locally advanced tumours.

! Patients at high risk of colorectal malignancy

- Patients with family history
- Familial polyposis
- Sporadic adenomatous polyps
- Inflammatory bowel disease

KEY POINTS

- Colorectal cancer is the second commonest malignancy in the UK.
- The Dukes' classification is used to stage the tumour after resection.

CASE 19: LOOSE STOOLS, WEIGHT LOSS AND RIGHT ILIAC FOSSA PAIN

History

A 33-year-old man presents to the surgical outpatient clinic complaining of increasing stool frequency (up to 5 times/day) for the past 4 months. His stool is looser than normal and occasionally contains mucus. His appetite has been healthy, but he has lost half a stone in weight. He also describes an intermittent colicky lower abdominal pain that occurs most days and is relieved by opening his bowels. He is otherwise well with no history of recent foreign travel. His father died at the age of 50 years from a colonic tumour.

Examination

The temperature is 37.5°C, the pulse rate is 90/min and the blood pressure is 130/70 mmHg. The right side of the abdomen is tender to deep palpation. No masses are palpable. Digital rectal examination is normal. Rigid sigmoidoscopy to 15 cm from the anal verge shows normal mucosa.

INVESTIGATIONS

		Normal
Haemoglobin	10.2 g/dL	11.5–16.0 g/dL
Mean cell volume	86 fL	76–96 fL
White cell count	6.0×10^9/L	$4.0–11.0 \times 10^9$/L
Platelets	232×10^9/L	$150–400 \times 10^9$/L
Sodium	145 mmol/L	135–145 mmol/L
Potassium	4.0 mmol/L	3.5–5.0 mmol/L
Urea	6.2 mmol/L	2.5–6.7 mmmol/L
Creatinine	79 μmol/L	44–80 μmol/L
C-reactive protein	98 mg/L	<5 mg/L

A colonoscopy is arranged and reveals injected, erythematous caecal and terminal ileal mucosa. A biopsy is taken and is reported as showing non-caseating granulomata with transmural inflammation of the bowel mucosa and frequent lymphoid aggregates in the subserosa.

Questions

- What is the diagnosis?
- What other intestinal manifestations of the disease are possible?
- What are the extra-intestinal manifestations of this disease?
- How is this condition treated medically?
- What are the indications for surgery?

ANSWER 19

Increasing frequency of stool, anorexia, low-grade fever, abdominal tenderness and anaemia suggest an inflammatory bowel disease. The histological findings are characteristic of Crohn's disease.

! Presentation of Crohn's disease

- Perforation of the affected bowel
- Stricturing of the bowel causing partial/complete obstruction
- Fistulation: e.g. enteroenteric, enterovesical, enteroureteric, enterocutaneous
- Uncontrollable haemorrhage (rare)

! Extra-intestinal manifestations of Crohn's

- Conjuntivitis and iritis
- Cirrhosis of the liver
- Cholangiocarcinoma
- Primary sclerosing cholangitis
- Renal stones and gallstones
- Erythema nodosum
- Pyoderma gangrenosum
- Psoriasis
- Ankylosing spondylitis

Potent anti-inflammatory drugs are the mainstay of medical therapy. Corticosteroids are used orally or intravenously. If the disease only affects the distal colon, topical (suppository/enema), steroids can be used. Salicylic acid derivatives (e.g. sulphasalazine) are used to control the disease and reduce the dose of steroids required to maintain remission. Other drugs used include anti-tumour necrosis factor alpha antibodies (e.g. infliximab) and immunosuppressive (e.g. methotrexate and azathioprine). Treatment with metronidazole can also help control symptoms.

! Indications for surgery

- Bowel perforation
- Massive haemorrhage
- Colonic dilatation
- Failure to respond to medical treatment
- Complicated fistulae
- Bowel stricturing and obstruction
- Failure to thrive in children

KEY POINTS

- Crohn's disease can affect any part of the bowel from the mouth to the anus.
- The initial management of uncomplicated Crohn's disease should be medical.

CASE 20: INCREASED BOWEL FREQUENCY AND RECTAL BLEEDING

History

A 40-year-old woman presents to the emergency department complaining of a 2-month history of bright rectal bleeding, motions up to six times per day and cramping lower abdominal pains. She has lost 2 stone in weight. She finished a course of Augmentin for a chest infection 2 weeks ago. She had an appendicectomy at the age of 16 years with no other past history of note. She visited Thailand on a family holiday 3 weeks ago.

Examination

The temperature is 37.5°C with a pulse rate of 98/min and a blood pressure of 140/70 mmHg. There is no lymphadenopathy. The abdomen is soft with tenderness to deep palpation in the left iliac fossa. Digital rectal examination shows soft stool with a small amount of bright red blood and mucus mixed in. Rigid sigmoidoscopy to 20 cm from the anal verge reveals bright red, friable rectal mucosa. A biopsy is taken.

INVESTIGATIONS

		Normal
Haemoglobin	13.2 g/dL	11.5–16.0 g/dL
Mean cell volume	86 fL	76–96 fL
White cell count	5.9×10^9/L	$4.0–11.0 \times 10^9$/L
Platelets	302×10^9/L	$150–400 \times 10^9$/L
Sodium	147 mmol/L	135–145 mmol/L
Potassium	4.8 mmol/L	3.5–5.0 mmol/L
Urea	6.9 mmol/L	2.5–6.7 mmmol/L
Creatinine	50 μmol/L	44–80 μmol/L
Amylase	68 IU/dL	0–100 IU/dL
Aspartate transaminase (AST)	32 IU/L	5–35 IU/L
Alkaline phosphatase (ALP)	74 IU/L	35–110 IU/L
Gamma-glutamyl transferase (GGT)	42 IU/L	11–51 IU/L
Albumin	37 g/L	35–50 g/L
Bilirubin	16 mmol/L	3–17 mmol/L
Erythrocyte sedimentation rate (ESR)	49 mm/h	1–13 mm/h

Questions

- What differential diagnoses would you consider?
- The biopsy suggests ulcerative colitis. What are the typical histological findings?
- How should the patient be managed acutely?
- What is the potential for malignant change associated with this condition?

ANSWER 20

! The main differential diagnoses for a patient with this history and symptoms

- *Inflammatory bowel disease*: Crohn's disease or ulcerative colitis
- *Infective diarrhoea: Shigella, Salmonella, Yersinia* and *Campylobacter*
- *Pseudomembranous colitis*: secondary to antibiotic use

In view of the patient's history, a biopsy of the rectal mucosa and stool sample should be sent. Microbiology can analyse the sample for an infective cause or test for *Clostridium difficile* toxin in cases of pseudomembranous colitis.

Ulcerative colitis occurs most commonly between the ages of 15 and 40 years, and usually involves the rectum then progresses more proximally. Typical histological changes include infiltration with acute and chronic inflammatory cells that is confined to the mucosa (unlike Crohn's disease where changes are transmural). In severe cases there is fissuring and transmural inflammation, making it difficult to distinguish Crohn's disease from ulcerative colitis on the basis of histology.

Medical management is aimed at controlling inflammation and reducing symptoms. In cases of severe colitis, nutritional support and correction of electrolyte disturbances may also be required. Corticosteroids can be used to induce remission, and salicylic acid derivatives employed to maintain remission – these can be administered as enemas or suppositories where the disease only involves the rectum. If diarrhoea is particularly problematic, agents such as codeine phosphate and loperamide may be considered.

The potential for malignant change is relatively high with long-standing ulcerative colitis and the risk in patients with pancolitis is approximately 3 per cent after 10 years. The risk of developing mucosal dysplasia increases with time, and surveillance should commence after 7 years. Colonoscopy and biopsy are performed every 2–3 years. If dysplasia is detected, the patient should undergo total colectomy with end ileostomy.

KEY POINTS

- Long-standing ulcerative colitis carries a ~3 per cent risk of malignant change after 10 years.
- Colonoscopy and biopsy are performed every 2–3 years.

UPPER GASTROINTESTINAL

CASE 21: RIGHT UPPER QUADRANT PAIN

History

A 44-year-old woman presented to the emergency department with a 1-day history of constant abdominal pain and vomiting. The pain came on suddenly, shortly after eating her evening meal. This was followed by intermittent bouts of bilious vomiting. She has diabetes and is concerned about her blood sugars as she has not been able to eat a normal diet since the pain started. Her bowels have opened normally and she has no urinary symptoms.

Examination

The patient is febrile with a temperature of 38°C and a pulse rate of 116/min. She is not clinically jaundiced. On examination of the abdomen, she is found to have tenderness in the right upper quadrant, which is worsened by placing two fingers beneath the tip of the ninth costal cartilage during inspiration. A tender mass is palpable in the right upper quadrant. The urine is clear and rectal examination is normal.

INVESTIGATIONS

		Normal
Haemoglobin	11.7 g/dL	11.5–16.0 g/dL
Mean cell volume	81 fL	76–96 fL
White cell count	18×10^9/L	$4.0–11.0 \times 10^9$/L
Platelets	312×10^9/L	$150–400 \times 10^9$/L
Sodium	135 mmol/L	135–145 mmol/L
Potassium	4.4 mmol/L	3.5–5.0 mmol/L
Urea	4 mmol/L	2.5–6.7 mmmol/L
Creatinine	69 μmol/L	44–80 μmol/L
Amylase	69 IU/dL	0–100 IU/dL
Aspartate transaminase (AST)	67 IU/dL	5–35 IU/L
Alkaline phosphatase (ALP)	76 IU/dL	35–110 IU/L
Gamma-glutamyl transferase (GGT)	50 IU/dL	11–51 IU/L
Albumin	42 g/L	35–50 g/L
Bilirubin	25 mmol/L	3–17 mmol/L
Blood glucose	27 mmol/L	3.5–5.5 mmol/L

Questions

- Whose sign is elicited on examination of the abdomen?
- What is the most likely diagnosis?
- What is your first-line treatment?
- What would you prescribe to treat the high blood glucose?
- What specific complication is this patient at risk of?

ANSWER 21

Murphy's sign has been demonstrated, which is described as tenderness under the tip of the ninth costal cartilage, which catches on inspiration. A palpable mass, caused by inflammation and adherent omentum, is present in up to 40 per cent of patients with cholecystitis. An abdominal ultrasound should be requested, which should confirm a thickened gallbladder wall with surrounding free fluid, supporting the diagnosis. Fifteen per cent of patients with acute cholecystitis may also be jaundiced. The majority of episodes of acute cholecystitis settle with analgesia and antibiotics. This patient's diabetes should be controlled with an insulin infusion, until she restarts a normal diet. For patients with recurrent episodes, or if the symptoms fail to settle despite conservative treatment, many centres now perform surgery during the same hospital admission. If this is not appropriate, then elective cholecystectomy can be carried out at an interval of approximately 6 weeks, after the inflammation has settled.

Acute cholecystitis can lead to a build up of infected bile within the gallbladder lumen, resulting in an empyema. The gallbladder can also become gangrenous, leading to perforation. Patients are at increased risk if they are diabetic, immunosuppressed, obese or have a haemoglobinopathy. Initial decompression may be accomplished under radiographic guidance or via intra-operative laparoscope-guided needle drainage. Elderly patients with significant comorbidities must be treated aggressively with antibiotics and early decompression, as the resulting sepsis can be life-threatening.

KEY POINT

- The majority of episodes of acute cholecystitis settle conservatively with analgesia and antibiotics.

CASE 22: EPIGASTRIC PAIN AND VOMITING

History

A 50-year-old man presents to the emergency department with vomiting and epigastric pain which radiates through to the back. The pain was of gradual onset, coming on over the last 2 days. He denies any previous episodes. He is not on any regular medication, but admits to drinking in excess of eight cans of lager a day. He is a heavy smoker, but denies any recreational drug use. He is homeless and relates his heavy drinking to depression.

Examination

The patient is sweaty and agitated. He says he is unable to lie flat for the examination and vomits persistently. His blood pressure is 150/80 mmHg and he has a pulse rate of 120/min. Palpation of his abdomen reveals tenderness in the epigastrium. The abdomen is not distended and he has normal bowel sounds. Rectal examination is unremarkable.

INVESTIGATIONS

		Normal
Haemoglobin	12 g/dL	11.5–16.0 g/dL
Mean cell volume	102 fL	76–96 fL
White cell count	13.3 × 10^9/L	4.0–11.0 × 10^9/L
Platelets	310 × 10^9/L	150–400 × 10^9/L
Sodium	132 mmol/L	135–145 mmol/L
Potassium	4.2 mmol/L	3.5–5.0 mmol/L
Urea	5 mmol/L	2.5–6.7 mmmol/L
Creatinine	72 μmol/L	44–80 μmol/L
Amylase	4672 IU/dL	0–100 IU/dL
Aspartate transaminase (AST)	30 IU/L	5–35 IU/L
Gamma-glutamyl transferase (GGT)	212 IU/L	11–51 IU/L
Albumin	25 g/L	35–50 g/L
Bilirubin	12 mmol/L	3–17 mmol/L
Glucose	5 mmol/L	3.5–5.5 mmol/L
Lactate dehydrogenase (LDH)	84 IU/L	70–250 IU/L
Total serum calcium	2.35 mmol/L	2.12–2.65 mmol/L

Questions

- What is the most likely diagnosis?
- Which important differential diagnosis should be excluded?
- How will you grade the severity of the condition?
- What are its causes?
- What are the other causes of the elevated serum marker of this condition?
- How will you manage the condition?
- Give four potential complications.

ANSWER 22

The most obvious abnormal result is the raised amylase, giving a diagnosis of acute pancreatitis. The history and macrocytosis would suggest this is of alcoholic aetiology, but it is important to ultrasound the abdomen to exclude gallstones as the cause. The pain is typically severe and radiates through to the back, due to the retroperitoneal position of the pancreas. Vomiting is also a common feature, as a result of gastric stasis caused by the local inflammation. The severity of the attack has no relation to the rise in serum amylase. Twenty per cent of cases of pancreatitis have a normal serum amylase, particularly when there is an alcoholic aetiology.

It is important to exclude a perforated peptic ulcer in this patient. This should be done with an erect chest X-ray, which would show free subphrenic air in 90 per cent of cases. The serum amylase can be elevated in a patient with gastric perforation due to the systemic absorption of pancreatic enzymes from the abdominal cavity. An amylase rise of over 1000 IU/dL, however, is usually diagnostic of acute pancreatitis.

Ranson's criteria are used to grade the severity of alcoholic pancreatitis, but it takes 48 h before the score can be used. Each fulfilled criterion scores a point and the total indicates the severity.

- *On admission*:
  - age >55 years
  - white cell count $>16 \times 10^9$ L
  - LDH >600 IU/L
  - AST >120 IU/L
  - glucose >10 mmol/L
  - fluid sequestration >6 L
- *Within 48 h*:
  - haematocrit fall >10 per cent
  - urea rise >0.9 mmol/L
  - calcium <2mmol/L
  - partial pressure of oxygen (po_2) <60 mmHg
  - base deficit >4

Estimates on mortality are based on the number of points scored: 0–2 = 2 per cent; 3–4 = 15 per cent; 5–6 = 40 per cent; >7 = 100 per cent.

! Causes of acute pancreatitis

- *Common* (80 per cent): gallstones, alcohol
- *Rare* (20 per cent): idiopathic, infection (mumps, coxsackie B virus), iatrogenic (endoscopic retrograde cholangiopancreatography [ERCP]), trauma, ampullary or pancreatic tumours, drugs (salicylates, azathioprine, cimetidine), pancreatic structural anomalies (pancreatic divisum), metabolic (hypertriglyceridaemia, raised Ca^{2+}), hypothermia

Causes of hyperamylasaemia

- Perforated peptic ulcer
- Mesenteric infarction
- Cholecystitis
- Generalized peritonitis
- Intestinal obstruction
- Ruptured ectopic pregnancy
- Diabetic ketoacidosis
- Liver failure
- Bowel perforation
- Renal failure
- Ruptured abdominal aortic aneurysm

The aim of treatment is to halt the progression of local inflammation into systemic inflammation, which can result in multi-organ failure. Patients will often require nursing on a high-dependency or intensive care unit. They require prompt fluid resuscitation, a urinary catheter and central venous pressure monitoring. Early enteral feeding is advocated by some specialists. If there is evidence of sepsis, the patient should receive broad-spectrum antibiotics. An ultrasound may demonstrate the presence of gallstones, biliary obstruction or a pseudocyst. Computerized tomography is used to confirm the diagnosis a few days after the onset of the symptoms, and can be used to assess for pancreatic necrosis.

Complications of pancreatitis

Local	*Systemic*
Pancreatic pseudocyst	Renal failure
Abscess formation	Respiratory failure
Biliary obstruction	Septic shock
Fistula formation	Electrolyte disturbance
Thrombosis	Multi-organ failure and death

KEY POINTS

- Ranson's criteria are used to grade the severity of acute alcoholic pancreatitis.
- Patients should be managed aggressively and may require treatment in a high-dependency unit or on intensive care.

CASE 23: FEVER, PAIN AND JAUNDICE

History

As the junior doctor on call, you are asked to review the blood results of an 87-year-old man, who was admitted that morning with possible appendicitis. He is confused and unable to give an accurate history. He had been spiking temperatures during the afternoon and had increasing right-sided abdominal pain.

Examination

The observation chart shows he has a temperature of 38°C and a tachycardia of 120/min. You notice he has a yellow discolouration of the skin and sclera, and abdominal examination reveals that the maximal tenderness is in the right upper quadrant. There are no palpable masses or abdominal herniae. Rectal examination demonstrates normal stool with no palpable rectal mass. A plain abdominal radiograph, done that morning, was normal.

INVESTIGATIONS

		Normal
Haemoglobin	15 g/dL	11.5–16.0 g/dL
Mean cell volume	82 fL	76–96 fL
White cell count	21×10^9/L	$4.0–11.0 \times 10^9$/L
Platelets	344×10^9/L	$150–400 \times 10^9$/L
Sodium	136 mmol/L	135–145 mmol/L
Potassium	4.5 mmol/L	3.5–5.0 mmol/L
Urea	6 mmol/L	2.5–6.7 mmmol/L
Creatinine	72 μmol/L	44–80 μmol/L
Amylase	69 IU/dL	0–100 IU/dL
Aspartate transaminase (AST)	68 IU/L	5–35 IU/L
Alkaline phosphatase (ALP)	442 IU/L	35–110 IU/L
Gamma-glutamyl transferase (GGT)	121 IU/L	11–51 IU/L
Bilirubin	92 mmol/L	3–17 mmol/L
Albumin	42 g/L	35–50 g/L
Blood glucose	4.0 mmol/L	3.5–5.5 mmol/L
C-reactive protein (CRP)	212 mg/L	0–6 mg/L

Questions

- What is the likely diagnosis?
- What are the classical characteristics to indicate this?
- What are the most common causes?
- Which are the most common organisms?
- How should the patient be managed?
- What investigations should be performed?

ANSWER 23

The collective symptoms of pain, jaundice and fever are known as Charcot's biliary triad and are characteristic of ascending cholangitis. Gallstones are the most common cause of acute cholangitis, followed by endoscopic retrograde cholangiopancreatography (ERCP) and tumours. The most common causative organisms are *Escherichia coli*, *Klebsiella*, *Enterobacter*, enterococci, and Group D streptococci.

Causes of ascending cholangitis

- Cholelithiasis
- ERCP
- Tumours: pancreatic, periampullary, cholangiocarcinoma

The patient needs intravenous fluid resuscitation and a urinary catheter, with strict hourly urine output measurements. Blood cultures should be taken on at least two separate occasions from two different sites, and broad-spectrum antibiotics should be commenced. Imaging studies are essential to confirm the presence and cause of the biliary obstruction and also help to rule out other conditions. Ultrasonography is the most commonly used initial imaging modality. Gallstones may not be directly visualized by ultrasound or computerized tomography (CT), so obstruction is diagnosed on the basis of the common bile duct (CBD) diameter. The upper limit of the normal diameter for the CBD is 5 mm. Greater than 7 mm indicates obstruction, although the bile duct diameter increases in the elderly and after cholecystectomy. If an obstruction of the CBD is confirmed, the patient should proceed to ERCP. The obstruction can then be relieved by removing the stone or inserting a biliary stent.

KEY POINTS

- Pain, fever and jaundice are classical features of ascending cholangitis.
- Gallstones are the most common cause.

CASE 24: SUDDEN-ONSET EPIGASTRIC PAIN

History

A 41-year-old businessman presents to the emergency department with epigastric pain and vomiting. The pain began suddenly 2 h previously, followed by 3–4 episodes of bilious vomiting. He had been previously fit and well. He is a smoker and drinks 40–60 units of alcohol per week.

Examination

The patient is sweaty and only comfortable while lying still. His blood pressure is 170/90 mmHg, pulse 110/min and temperature 37.5°C. The upper abdomen is tender and rigid on palpation.

INVESTIGATIONS

		Normal
Haemoglobin	12.0 g/dL	11.5–16.0 g/dL
Mean cell volume	86 fL	76–96 fL
White cell count	13.2×10^9/L	$4.0–11.0 \times 10^9$/L
Platelets	250×10^9/L	$150–400 \times 10^9$/L
Sodium	137 mmol/L	135–145 mmol/L
Potassium	3.5 mmol/L	3.5–5.0 mmol/L
Urea	5 mmol/L	2.5–6.7 mmmol/L
Creatinine	62 μmol/L	44–80 μmol/L
Amylase	250 IU/dL	0–100 IU/dL
Aspartate transaminase (AST)	30 IU/L	5–35 IU/L
Gamma-glutamyl transferase (GGT)	242 IU/L	11–51 IU/L
Albumin	45 g/L	35–50 g/L
Bilirubin	12 mmol/L	3–17 mmol/L
Glucose	5 mmol/L	3.5–5.5 mmol/L
Lactate dehydrogenase (LDH)	84 IU/L	70–250 IU/L
Total serum calcium	2.35 mmol/L	2.12–2.65 mmol/L

Figure 24.1 shows an erect chest X-ray.

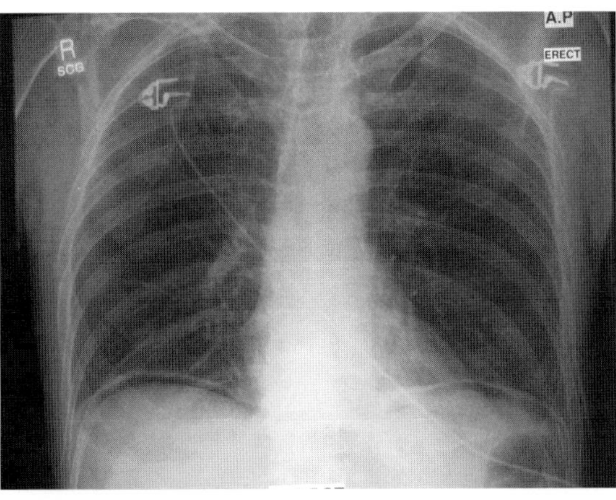

Figure 24.1 Erect chest X-ray.

Questions

- What is the likely diagnosis?
- How should this patient be managed?
- How should this patient be managed after discharge?

ANSWER 24

The X-ray shows free intraperitoneal gas beneath the hemidiaphragms, consistent with a perforated intra-abdominal viscus.

The most common cause is a perforation of a peptic ulcer. Ulcers situated on the anterior duodenal wall perforate into the abdominal cavity resulting in free intraperitoneal gas. Posteriorly, ulcers erode into the gastroduodenal artery, which is more likely to result in bleeding.

! Common causes of a pneumoperitoneum

- *Ruptured hollow viscus*: perforated peptic ulcer or diverticulum, necrotizing enterocolitis, toxic megacolon, inflammatory bowel disease
- *Infection*: infection of the peritoneal cavity with gas-forming organisms and/or rupture of an adjacent abscess
- *Iatrogenic factors*: recent abdominal surgery, abdominal trauma, a leaking surgical anastomosis, misplaced chest drain, endoscopic perforation

It is important to be sure that the chest X-ray is taken in the erect position. However, 10 per cent of perforations will still not demonstrate free gas on an erect chest X-ray. A lateral decubitus radiograph can be taken if the diagnosis is unclear. If there is any diagnostic doubt then water-soluble contrast or computerized tomography (CT) may confirm the presence of a perforation.

The patient requires prompt fluid resuscitation, with central venous pressure monitoring and hourly urine output measurements. Nasogastric intubation, broad-spectrum antibiotics and analgesia should also be given. Most patients require surgery after appropriate resuscitation. Conservative management may be considered if there is significant comorbidity. Postoperatively, patients should receive *Helicobacter pylori* eradication therapy and should continue on a proton pump inhibitor.

The recommended weekly intake of alcohol is <28 units per week for males and <21 = units for females. He will require follow-up with his general practitioner to help modify his lifestyle to prevent relapse.

KEY POINT

- Pneumoperitoneum is not evident on erect an chest X-ray in 10 per cent of cases.

CASE 25: ABDOMINAL TRAUMA

History

You are called urgently to the resuscitation room for a trauma call. An 18-year-old girl has fallen from her horse. During her descent the horse kicked her, and she is now complaining of generalized abdominal pain and left shoulder-tip pain.

Examination

She is talking and examination of her chest is normal. The oxygen saturations are 100 per cent on 24 per cent oxygen. Initially, her pulse rate is 110/min with a blood pressure of 84/60 mmHg. She is slightly drowsy and her Glasgow Coma Score (GCS) is 14. On examination of the abdomen, there is an abrasion on the left side beneath the costal margin with tenderness in the left upper quadrant. There is no evidence of any other injuries and the urinalysis is clear. The patient is given 2 L of intravenous fluids and the blood pressure improves to 130/90 mmHg. As the patient has now become stable, a computerized tomography scan (CT) of the chest and abdomen is obtained. The CT image is shown in Fig. 25.1.

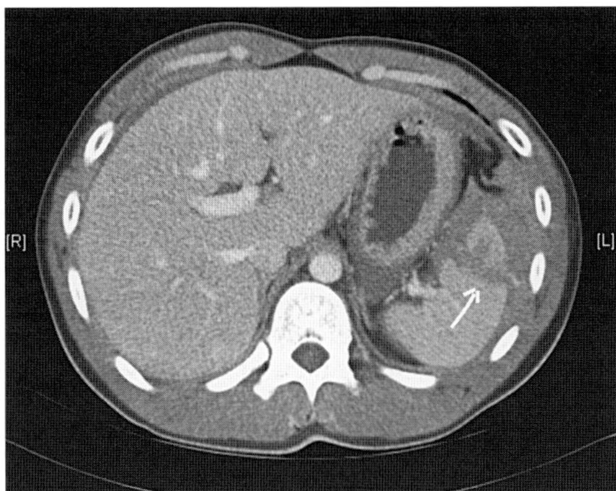

Figure 25.1 Computerized tomography of the abdomen.

On returning to the emergency department the patient becomes increasingly agitated. The nurse informs you that her blood pressure is now 80/60 mmHg and the pulse rate is 130/min.

Questions

- What does the CT show?
- Are there any alternative investigations to CT?
- What special requirements may this patient have postoperatively?

ANSWER 25

The patient has sustained a tear to the splenic capsule causing intraperitoneal bleeding. The CT shows the fractured spleen with surrounding haematoma. The shoulder-tip pain described is known as Kehr's sign, and is indicative of blood in the peritoneal cavity causing diaphragmatic irritation. Unstable patients suspected of splenic injury and intra-abdominal haemorrhage should undergo exploratory laparotomy and splenic repair or removal. Blunt trauma, with evidence of haemodynamic instability which is unresponsive to fluid challenge, should be considered to be a life-threatening solid organ (splenic) injury. Those patients who respond to an initial fluid bolus, only to deteriorate again with a drop in blood pressure and increasing tachycardia, are also likely to have a solid organ injury with ongoing haemorrhage. Transfer to the CT scanner can be extremely dangerous for an unstable patient.

Focused abdominal sonographic technique (FAST) is helpful in diagnosing the presence or absence of blood in the peritoneal cavity. Diagnostic peritoneal lavage may be a valuable adjunct if time permits and multiple other injuries are present. In a haemodynamically stable trauma patient, CT scanning provides an ideal non-invasive method for evaluating the spleen. The decision for operative intervention is determined by the grade of the injury and the patient's current or pre-existing medical conditions. If possible, it is preferable to repair minor tears of the spleen. Those patients who undergo splenectomy have a lifetime risk of septicaemia and should receive immunizations against *pneumococcus*, *haemophilus* and *meningococcus*.

KEY POINTS

- Whenever possible the spleen should be conserved.
- Patients require lifelong prophylactic antibiotics after splenectomy.

CASE 26: HEPATOMEGALY

History

A general practitioner refers an 87-year-old woman to the surgical outpatient department. The patient has had a 6-week history of constant right-sided abdominal pain which radiates up under the ribs and into her right shoulder. There are no relieving or exacerbating factors. She was fit and well up until 4 years ago, when she had a right hemicolectomy for a Dukes' B caecal adenocarcinoma. She did not receive any chemoradiotherapy postoperatively and there was no evidence of metastatic disease at the time of her operation. Recently, she feels she has lost weight and has felt tired. She describes no recent change in her bowel habit or rectal bleeding.

Examination

There is no evidence of pallor, jaundice, clubbing or lymphadenopathy. The chest is clear and heart sounds are normal. Examination of the abdomen reveals a palpable irregular liver border about 3 cm below the costal margin. There are no other palpable masses in the abdomen and digital rectal examination is normal.

INVESTIGATIONS

In view of this woman's history, a computerized tomography (CT) of the abdomen is organized (Fig. 26.1).

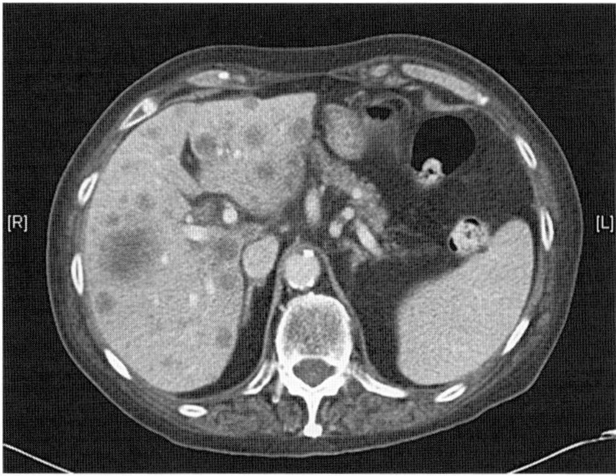

Figure 26.1 Computerized tomography of the abdomen.

Questions

- What does the CT show?
- What investigation would confirm the diagnosis in this patient?
- Give six other causes of hepatomegaly.
- What are the options for managing this patient?

ANSWER 26

The CT shows metastatic deposits within the liver. It is likely this is recurrent disease after her previous colonic resection. A CT-guided biopsy would confirm the possible origin of these lesions.

! Causes of hepatomegaly

Smooth generalized enlargement

- Hepatitis
- Congestive cardiac failure
- Micronodular cirrhosis
- Hepatic vein obstruction (Budd–Chiari syndrome)
- Amyloidosis

Craggy generalized enlargement

- Metastatic secondaries
- Macronodular cirrhosis

Localized swelling

- Hepatocellular carcinoma
- Riedel's lobe
- Hydatid cyst
- Liver abscess

A CT scan may demonstrate recurrence of the bowel malignancy. Tumour markers may be raised, and a CT-guided biopsy of the liver deposits may confirm the source of the recurrence. It is important to send a full blood count as she has been feeling tired recently and may be anaemic. The patient should be brought back to the clinic, with her relatives, to discuss the options for further management. The number of metastases in the liver and their distribution would make local resection unfeasible. Chemotherapy may be discussed, but may not be appropriate in this patient. It is unlikely to prolong the patient's life significantly and indeed may worsen her quality of life. The most important factor is to control the patient's pain. A palliative care team should be involved in her continued management.

KEY POINT

- Liver metastases can be surgically resected depending on their number and anatomical distribution.

CASE 27: LONG-STANDING GASTRO-OESOPHAGEAL REFLUX

History

A 60-year-old retired plumber is referred to the endoscopy unit by his general practitioner (GP). He has been suffering from heartburn for 5 years and is now complaining of difficulty in swallowing. He says he has to chew his food more than he used to and finds it difficult to eat meats. Despite this, he denies any weight loss and feels well in himself. He enjoys red wine and has a couple of glasses each evening. He has been a heavy smoker for about 40 years. He has not been to his GP before, as he thought the heartburn was probably related to his smoking. He is now concerned about his difficulty in swallowing.

Examination

There are no abnormal physical signs on full examination. An oesophagogastroduodenoscopy (OGD) is performed and a picture is taken (Fig. 27.1).

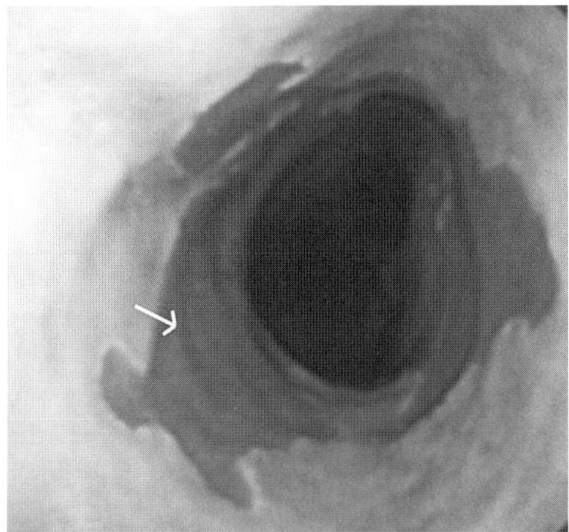

Figure 27.1 Distal oesophagus at endoscopy.

INVESTIGATIONS

		Normal
Haemoglobin	11.9 g/dL	11.5–16.0 g/dL
Mean cell volume	86 fL	76–96 fL
White cell count	10×10^9/L	$4.0–11.0 \times 10^9$/L
Platelets	252×10^9/L	$150–400 \times 10^9$/L
Sodium	137 mmol/L	135–145 mmol/L
Potassium	4.2 mmol/L	3.5–5.0 mmol/L
Urea	5.0 mmol/L	2.5–6.7 mmmol/L
Creatinine	62 μmol/L	44–80 μmol/L

Questions

- What does this investigation show?
- What are the histological changes to the lower oesophagus?
- What are the possible causes of this patient's dysphagia?
- Does the patient require any follow-up?

ANSWER 27

The endoscopy reveals that as a result of prolonged acid reflux, the normal squamous mucosa of the oesophagus has undergone metaplastic change leading to caudal migration of the squamocolumnar junction (arrow in Fig. 27.1). This is known as Barrett's oesophagus.

Approximately one-third of patients with Barrett's oesophagus develop a peptic stricture. Peptic strictures usually present with a gradual onset of dysphagia to solids, and could be the cause of this patient's recent symptoms. Symptoms of heartburn and regurgitation may improve as a stricture develops and provides a barrier to further episodes of reflux. Treatment should be initially by dilatation, followed by medical or surgical treatment of the underlying reflux disease. Even small degrees of luminal dilatation can produce significant improvements in symptoms. Proton pump inhibitors are effective in reducing stricture recurrence and in the treatment of Barrett's oesophagus. If frequent dilatations are required despite acid suppression, then surgery should be considered.

The intestinal metaplasia of the distal oesophageal mucosa can progress to dysplasia and adenocarcinoma. The risk of cancer is increased by up to 30 times in patients with Barrett's oesophagus. If Barrett's oesophagus is found at endoscopy, then the patient should be started on lifelong acid suppression. The patient should then have endoscopic surveillance to detect dysplasia before progression to carcinoma.

! Causes of dysphagia

Outside the wall	*In the wall*	*Within the lumen*
Lymph nodes	Oesophagitis	Foreign body
Goitre	Stricture	Oesophageal web
Enlarged left atrium	Motility disorders, e.g. achalasia, bulbar palsy	
Lung cancer	Malignancy	
Thoracic aneurysms	Scleroderma	
Pharyngeal pouch		

KEY POINTS

- Up to 10 per cent of patients with long-standing gastro-oesophageal reflux develop a peptic stricture.
- If Barrett's oesophagus is found at endoscopy, then the patient should have regular endoscopic surveillance to screen for dysplasia.

CASE 28: DIFFICULTY IN SWALLOWING

History

A 79-year-old man is admitted from the endoscopy unit after an oesophagogastroscopy. He initially presented to his general practitioner with increasing difficulty in swallowing. Over the preceding months he has required a soft diet and is now only able to tolerate thin fluids. These symptoms have been associated with a weight loss of 1 stone over the last month. He is a heavy smoker and enjoys a half bottle of wine each evening. He has no other relevant past medical history.

Examination

The patient is cachexic in appearance. The endoscopic finding is shown in Fig. 28.1.

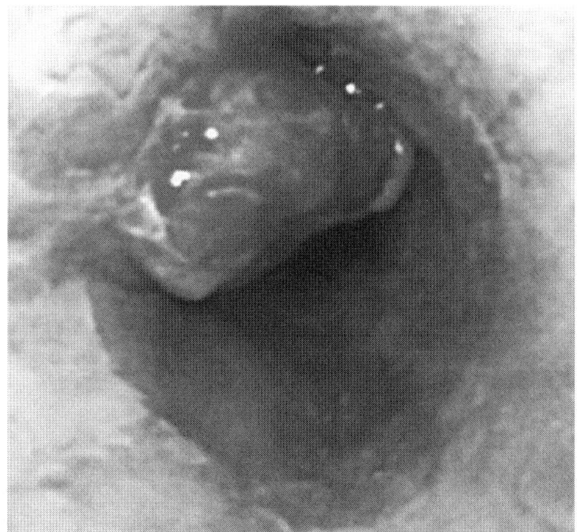

Figure 28.1 Distal oesophagus at endoscopy.

INVESTIGATIONS

		Normal
Haemoglobin	14.0 g/dL	11.5–16.0 g/dL
Mean cell volume	86 fL	76–96 fL
White cell count	7.2×10^9/L	$4.0–11.0 \times 10^9$/L
Platelets	360×10^9/L	$150–400 \times 10^9$/L
Sodium	142 mmol/L	135–145 mmol/L
Potassium	4.3 mmol/L	3.5–5.0 mmol/L
Urea	4 mmol/L	2.5–6.7 mmmol/L
Creatinine	62 μmol/L	44–80 μmol/L

Questions

- What is the likely diagnosis?
- What are the risk factors?
- How should the patient be staged?
- What are the therapeutic options?

ANSWER 28

This patient has an oesophageal carcinoma. It typically affects patients between 60 and 70 years of age and has a higher incidence in males. Worldwide, squamous cell carcinomas account for up to 90 per cent of all oesophageal cancers. In the UK and USA, over half of the new presentations are now adenocarcinomas. It is thought this is because of the increased incidence of Barrett's metaplasia, as a consequence of gastro-oesophageal reflux disease. Dysphagia is the most common presenting symptom and is often associated with weight loss. Patients can also present with bleeding or with respiratory symptoms due to aspiration or fistulation of the tumour into the respiratory tract.

! Risk factors for oesophageal carcinoma

- Alcohol and smoking
- Nitrosamines and aflatoxins
- Deficiency of vitamins A and C
- Achalasia
- Coeliac disease
- Tylosis
- *Barrett's oesophagus*: adenocarcinoma

Staging should by computerized tomography (CT) of the chest and abdomen (Fig. 28.2). If this reveals metastatic disease then no further assessment for operability is required. If the patient is fit for surgery, the tumour depth and lymph node involvement should be assessed by endoscopic ultrasound. Approximately 40 per cent of patients are suitable for surgical resection. The surgical procedure should aim for complete tumour removal (macroscopic and microscopic) and a regional lymph node clearance. Clear resectional margins and the lymph node status are important prognostic indicators. Postoperative chemotherapy or radiotherapy for node-positive patients has produced improvements in survival. Neoadjuvant therapy to downstage the tumours prior to resection is now carried out in many centres and is still being evaluated.

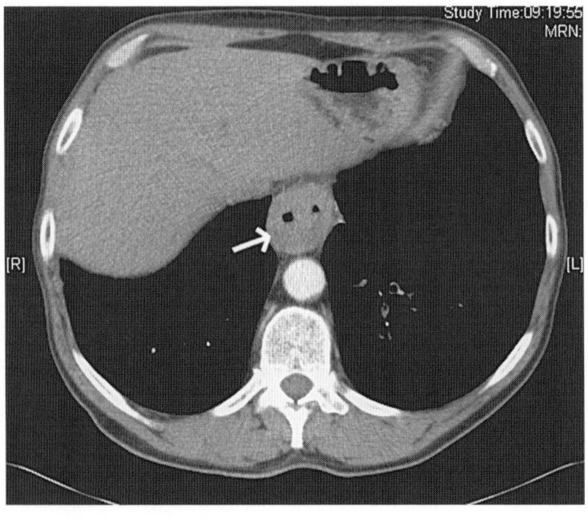

Figure 28.2 Computerized tomography showing oesophageal thickening as a result of oesophageal cancer (arrow). No liver metastases are seen.

For patients with unresectable tumours the aim is to relieve dysphagia with minimal risks. This can be achieved by repeated dilatations or tumour ablation using a laser. Radiotherapy can also reduce pain and improve swallowing difficulties. Currently an increasing number of patients are being treated by endoscopic or radiological placement of self-expanding stents. The complications of stents include oesophageal perforation, migration and blockage from ingrowth by the tumour.

KEY POINTS

- The incidence of oesophageal adenocarcinoma is increasing.
- The use of oesophageal stents has improved palliation in patients with unresectable disease.

CASE 29: PAINLESS JAUNDICE

History

A 73-year-old man is admitted from surgical outpatients. You have been asked to clerk the patient and initiate his investigations. For the last 3 months, he has noticed a progressively deepening yellow discolouration of his skin. He has not had any abdominal pain. His appetite has reduced significantly and he has found that his clothes have become loose. He has also noticed that his urine has darkened and his stools have become pale and difficult to flush. He enjoys the occasional whisky at home in the evening and has smoked 10 cigarettes a day since he was a teenager. He is not on any regular medication.

Examination

The patient appears underweight and has a yellow discolouration of the skin and sclera. The heart sounds are normal with a blood pressure of 136/64 mmHg and a pulse of 86/min. He is afebrile and his chest is clear. The abdomen is soft with a smooth mass present in the right upper quadrant, which moves with respiration.

INVESTIGATIONS

		Normal
Haemoglobin	13.0 g/dL	11.5–16.0 g/dL
Mean cell volume	86 fL	76–96 fL
White cell count	12 × 10^9/L	4.0–11.0 × 10^9/L
Platelets	260 × 10^9/L	150–400 × 10^9/L
Sodium	137 mmol/L	135–145 mmol/L
Potassium	4.3 mmol/L	3.5–5.0 mmol/L
Urea	5 mmol/L	2.5–6.7 mmmol/L
Creatinine	65 μmol/L	44–80 μmol/L
Amylase	32 IU/L	0–100 IU/dL
Alkaline phosphatase (ALP)	229 IU/L	35–110 IU/L
Aspartate transaminase (AST)	96 IU/L	5–35 IU/L
Gamma-glutamyl transferase (GGT)	63 IU/L	11–51 IU/L
Albumin	46 g/L	35–50 g/L
Bilirubin	82 mmol/L	3–17 mmol/L
Glucose	5 mmol/L	3.5–5.5 mmol/L

Questions

- Why are the stools pale?
- What is Courvoisier's law?
- What additional investigations are required to make the diagnosis?
- How should this patient be managed?

ANSWER 29

The most likely cause in this patient is pancreatic cancer. The patient reports having pale floating stools, which is consistent with steatorrhoea caused by an inability to absorb fat from the digestive tract resulting in excess fat in the stools. Courvoisier's law states that a palpable gallbladder in the presence of jaundice, is unlikely to be secondary to gallstones. The presence of gallstones leads to a shrunken fibrotic gallbladder and is usually associated with pain. Pancreatic cancer classically presents with painless jaundice from biliary obstruction at the head of the pancreas and is associated with a distended gallbladder. Patients with pancreatic cancer can also present with epigastric pain, radiating through to the back, and vomiting due to duodenal obstruction.

Pancreatic cancer occurs in patients between 60 and 80 years of age, with a higher incidence in males than females. It is associated with chronic pancreatitis and smoking. The majority are adenocarcinomas and occur in the head of the pancreas. Roughly three-quarters have metastases at presentation, which is responsible for the very poor overall 5-year survival rate of less than 5 per cent. Ca 19-9 is the most useful tumour marker for pancreatic cancer with a sensitivity of 80 per cent and a specificity of 75 per cent. Abdominal ultrasound has a sensitivity of about 80 per cent for the detection of pancreatic cancer and excludes gallstones. Spiral computerized tomography (CT) has a sensitivity of greater than 90 per cent for detecting pancreatic tumours. Endoscopic ultrasound is now being used more frequently to stage tumours and is especially useful in periampullary tumours. Endoscopic retrograde cholangiopancreatography (ERCP) can be used to aid diagnosis, but is often reserved for therapeutic intervention.

Resectability of the tumour depends on the tumour size, whether the tumour invades the superior mesenteric artery or portal vein, the presence of ascites or the presence of nodal, peritoneal or liver metastases. Both ultrasound scan and CT often fail to detect small (<2 cm) metastases, so laparoscopy is used to identify liver or peritoneal disease. Laparoscopy detects metastases in about a quarter of patients who are negative after conventional imaging.

Only 15 per cent of tumours are resectable by pancreatic–duodenal resection (Whipple's operation). Operative mortality is reported to be less than 5 per cent, with a 5-year survival of approximately 35 per cent. Patients have a high incidence of postoperative morbidity, with a significant proportion becoming diabetic or requiring pancreatic supplementation.

The majority of patients are not suitable for resection. These patients require endoscopic stenting to relieve the bile duct obstruction. Duodenal obstruction can be relieved with a bypass procedure (gastrojejunostomy).

KEY POINT

- Only approximately 15 per cent of pancreatic malignancies are surgically resectable.

CASE 30: INTERMITTENT ABDOMINAL PAIN

History

A 50-year-old woman was referred to the surgical outpatient clinic by her general practitioner (GP). She had been complaining of intermittent bouts of abdominal pain over the preceding 6 months. When the pain occurred, it was constant, associated with nausea and usually lasted for a couple of hours. She had also noticed that fried foods triggered the attacks. In the referral letter, the GP also mentioned that her body mass index (BMI) was 38 but that she had been actively trying to lose weight. She has no past medical history and has recently been started on hormone-replacement therapy.

Examination

On examination, the patient is afebrile with a pulse rate of 80/min. She has no evidence of jaundice and no palpable lymphadenopathy. On palpation of her abdomen there is mild tenderness in the right upper quadrant. Rectal examination is normal and urinalysis is clear.

INVESTIGATIONS

		Normal
Haemoglobin	12 g/dL	11.5–16.0 g/dL
Mean cell volume	80 fL	76–96 fL
White cell count	11.0×10^9/L	$4.0–11.0 \times 10^9$/L
Platelets	315×10^9/L	$150–400 \times 10^9$/L
Sodium	137 mmol/L	135–145 mmol/L
Potassium	4.2 mmol/L	3.5–5.0 mmol/L
Urea	5.0 mmol/L	2.5–6.7 mmmol/L
Creatinine	77 μmol/L	44–80 μmol/L
Amylase	72 IU/dL	0–100 IU/dL
Alkaline phosphatase (ALP)	69 IU/L	35–110 IU/L
Aspartate transaminase (AST)	30 IU/L	5–35 IU/L
Gamma-glutamyl transferase (GGT)	45 IU/L	11–51 IU/L
Albumin	45 g/L	35–50 g/L
Bilirubin	12 mmol/L	3–17 mmol/L

Questions

- Which radiological investigation should be ordered and what might it show?
- What advice would you give the patient?
- What are the next steps in the management of this patient?

ANSWER 30

The history suggests a diagnosis of chronic cholecystitis or biliary colic. An ultrasound of the abdomen should be requested, which may reveal gallstones situated within a thick-walled gallbladder (arrow in Fig. 30.1).

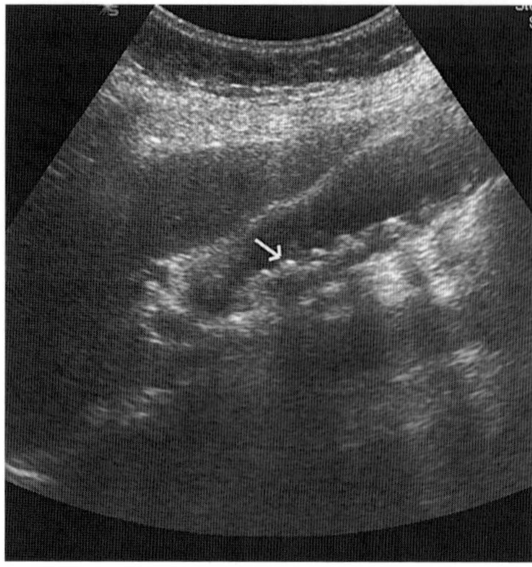

Figure 30.1 Ultrasonography showing multiple calculi within the gallbladder (arrow).

Gallstones are present in up to 10 per cent of females in their 40s and are less common in males. Typically, they are believed to be more common in 'fair, fat, fertile females of forty', but in fact can occur in any individual. Impaction of a gallstone in the gallbladder outlet causes contraction of the smooth muscle leading to pain. It is usually continuous and may radiate to the lower pole of the right scapula.

Biliary colic is the presenting symptom in over 80 per cent of patients with gallstones. More than two-thirds of those patients have a second episode within 2 years. If the pain persists or the patient becomes febrile, then the patient may have developed cholecystitis. This occurs when the gallstones remain impacted in the gallbladder outlet, leading to inflammation of the gallbladder wall.

Initially, patients are advised to avoid high-fat meals, although there is little evidence to show that this reduces further attacks. Laparoscopic cholecystectomy should be offered to patients with persistent symptoms.

Patients with cholesterol gallstones can be offered treatment with ursodeoxycholic acid. This drug aims to dissolve the gallstones. Dissolution typically takes between 6 and 18 months and is only successful with small, purely cholesterol stones. Patients remain at risk of gallstone complications throughout this time, and treatment fails in many cases. After treatment, most patients will form new gallstones over the subsequent 5–10 years.

KEY POINTS

- Gallstones are present in 10 per cent of females in their 40s.
- The majority of gallstones remain symptomless.

CASE 31: POSTOPERATIVE CONFUSION

History

As the junior doctor on call, you are asked to review a 75-year-old woman who has become confused on the ward. She is 5 days post an emergency femoral hernia repair. The operation was straightforward and there are no complications from the surgery. Her past medical history includes osteoarthritis of her right knee, for which she is taking diclofenac. She is a non-smoker and drinks two units of alcohol per week. She lives on her own with no support from social services.

Examination

She is disorientated in time, place and person. You notice that she is pale and tachypnoeic. Her blood pressure is 90/70 mmHg with a pulse rate of 110/min. Her chest is clear with oxygen saturations of 97 per cent on air. On palpation of her abdomen, you note vague upper abdominal tenderness. Bowel sounds are present and the urinalysis is clear. The wound site is clean and there is no evidence of a haematoma.

INVESTIGATIONS

		Normal
Haemoglobin (Hb)	6.2 g/dL	11.5–16.0 g/dL
Mean cell volume	86 fL	76–96 fL
White cell count	9×10^9/L	$4.0–11.0 \times 10^9$/L
Platelets	250×10^9/L	$150–400 \times 10^9$/L
Sodium	132 mmol/L	135–145 mmol/L
Potassium	3.5 mmol/L	3.5–5.0 mmol/L
Urea	16 mmol/L	2.5–6.7 mmmol/L
Creatinine	79 μmol/L	44–80 μmol/L

Electrocardiogram shows sinus tachycardia.

Questions

- What are the most common causes of postoperative confusion?
- What is the most likely diagnosis in this patient?
- What are the common causes?
- Which further clinical examination would you perform to help confirm this?
- How would you manage this patient?

ANSWER 31

Postoperative confusion is common in surgical patients. Causes include infection (urinary tract, chest, wound sepsis) myocardial infarction, pulmonary embolism, opiate medication and alcohol withdrawal. In this case, it is most likely that the patient has become confused as a result of acute blood loss. The stress from her recent emergency surgery and the non-steroidal anti-inflammatory (NSAID) medication has resulted in an upper gastrointestinal bleed.

A rectal examination is an important part of the clinical assessment. The presence of melaena on the glove would indicate an upper gastrointestinal source of bleeding. Melaena is abnormally dark tarry faeces caused by the action of stomach acid on blood. The normocytic anaemia (Hb 6.2 g/dL) shows that a large acute bleed has occurred. The rise in urea (16 mmol/L) indicates protein absorption from blood in the gastrointestinal tract. A systolic blood pressure of 90 mmHg and tachycardia suggest the patient is in hypovolaemic shock and requires urgent resuscitation.

! Causes of upper gastrointestinal bleeding

- Duodenal/gastric ulcer
- Gastritis/gastric erosions
- Mallory–Weiss tear
- Duodenitis
- Oesophageal varices
- Gastrointestinal tract malignancy
- Medication (NSAIDS, steroids)

! Acute management of a gastrointestinal bleed

1 Protect airway and administer high-flow oxygen.
2 Insert two large-bore (14–16G) cannulae and take blood for full blood count, renal function, liver function, clotting and crossmatch 4–6 units.
3 Replace fluid, until blood is available.
4 Insert a urinary catheter and a central venous line with strict fluid balance monitoring.
5 Transfer to an appropriate level of care, i.e. a high-dependency unit.
6 Arrange an urgent endoscopy: less than 24 h if stable, immediate if unstable despite appropriate resuscitation.
7 If you suspect variceal bleeding (signs chronic liver disease or previous variceal bleed) then perform endoscopy within 4 h.
8 Start high-dose intravenous proton pump inhibitor.

KEY POINTS

- NSAIDs should be used cautiously in the elderly.
- Patients with bleeding peptic ulcers should have a repeat endoscopy to check the ulcer has healed and to exclude underlying malignancy.

CASE 32: CHRONIC EPIGASTRIC PAIN

History

A 50-year-old man is referred to the surgical outpatients with a 6-month history of epigastric pain, weight loss and altered bowel habit. The epigastric pain is present throughout the day and is not relieved by food. He has noticed that his bowels have been opening more frequently and that the stools are bulky, pale and malodorous. His appetite has been poor over the last couple of months and he has lost 2 stone in weight. His previous medical history includes treatment for alcohol dependence. He still drinks at least 10 units of alcohol per day and is a heavy smoker. Prior to his referral, the general practitioner organized an oesophagogastroduodenoscopy and ultrasound of the abdomen, both of which were normal.

Examination

The patient is pale, thin and unkempt. There is no jaundice or supraclavicular lymphadenopathy. The abdomen is soft and non-tender with no palpable masses or organomegaly. The patient has previously had a plain abdominal film which is shown in Fig. 32.1.

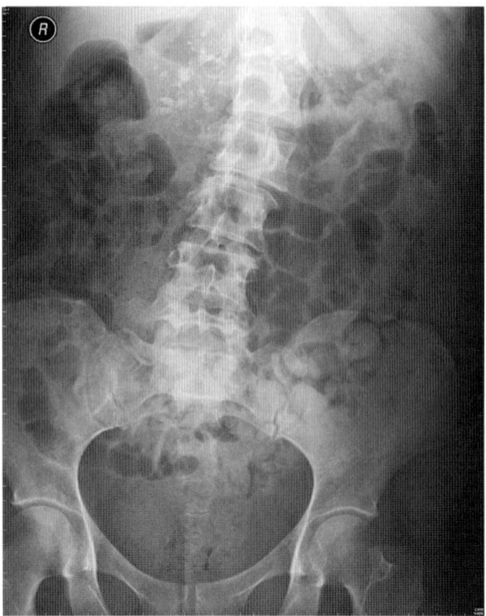

Figure 32.1 Plain X-ray of the abdomen.

INVESTIGATIONS

		Normal
Haemoglobin	13.0 g/dL	11.5–16.0 g/dL
Mean cell volume	108 fL	76–96 fL
White cell count	10×10^9/L	$4.0–11.0 \times 10^9$/L
Platelets	210×10^9/L	$150–400 \times 10^9$/L
Sodium	137 mmol/L	135–145 mmol/L
Potassium	3.6 mmol/L	3.5–5.0 mmol/L
Urea	6 mmol/L	2.5–6.7 mmmol/L
Creatinine	112 μmol/L	44–80 μmol/L
Amylase	222 IU/dL	0–100 IU/dL
Aspartate transaminase (AST)	30 IU/dL	5–35 IU/L
Gamma-glutamyl transferase (GGT)	235 IU/L	11–51 IU/L
Albumin	32 g/L	35–50 g/L
Bilirubin	12 mmol/L	3–17 mmol/L
Glucose	12 mmol/L	3.5–5.5 mmol/L
Total serum calcium	2.36 mmol/L	2.12–2.65 mmol/L

Questions

- What does the X-ray show?
- What is the likely diagnosis?
- What are the common causes?
- What investigations are required to confirm the diagnosis?
- How should the patient be managed?

ANSWER 32

The patient has chronic pancreatitis. The X-ray demonstrates pancreatic calcification (arrow in Fig. 32.2).

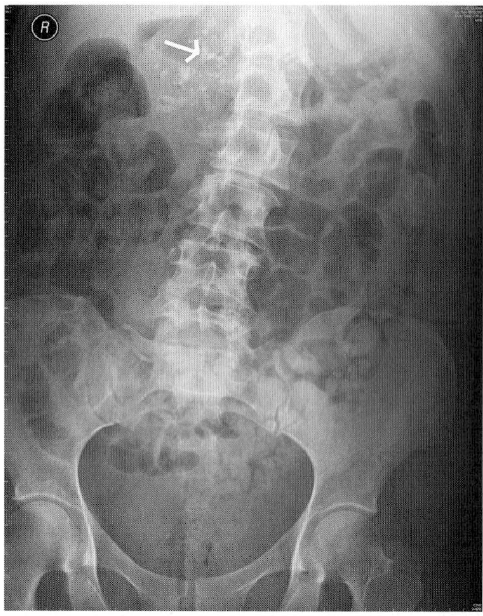

Figure 32.2 Plain X-ray of the abdomen. Arrow shows pancreatic calcification.

Chronic pancreatitis is an irreversible inflammation causing pancreatic fibrosis and calcification. Patients usually present with chronic abdominal pain and normal or mildly elevated pancreatic enzyme levels. The pancreas may have lost its endocrine and exocrine function, leading to diabetes mellitus and steatorrhea.

! Causes of chronic pancreatitis

- *Alcohol dependence*: most common cause
- *Idiopathic*: approximately 30 per cent
- *Cholelithiasis*: this is the most common cause of acute pancreatitis, but it is associated with chronic pancreatitis in less than 25 per cent of cases
- *Pancreatic duct strictures*
- *Pancreatic trauma*
- *Hereditary pancreatitis*: mutations in the gene for cationic trypsinogen on chromosome 7 appear to be involved in 60–75 per cent of cases of hereditary pancreatitis
- *Recurrent acute pancreatitis*
- *Cystic fibrosis*: an autosomal recessive disorder accounting for a small percentage of patients with chronic pancreatitis
- *Congenital causes*: pancreas divisum can cause chronic pancreatitis, although this is rare
- *Autoimmune disorders*: Sjögren's syndrome, primary biliary cirrhosis, and renal tubular acidosis
- *Other conditions*: hyperlipidaemia, hyperparathyroidism, and uraemia can cause chronic pancreatitis

Diagnostic studies may be normal in the early stages of chronic pancreatitis. The inflammatory changes can only be diagnosed on histological analysis of a biopsy. The mean age of onset is 40 years, with a male preponderance of 4:1. Pancreatic calcification is observed in approximately one-third of plain X-rays of patients with chronic pancreatitis (arrow in Fig. 32.2). Endoscopic retrograde cholangiopancreatography (ERCP) provides the most accurate visualization of the pancreatic ductal system and has been regarded as essential for diagnosing chronic pancreatitis. One limitation of ERCP is that it cannot be used to evaluate the pancreatic parenchyma, and histologically proven chronic pancreatitis can be found after a normal ERCP. Magnetic resonance cholangiopancreatography (MRCP) imaging provides information on the pancreatic parenchyma and adjacent abdominal viscera. Pancreatic function tests can provide useful information using the serum trypsin or faecal fat levels.

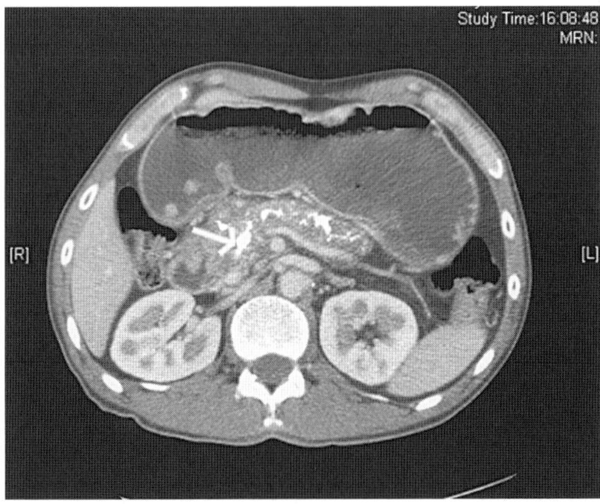

Figure 32.3 Computerized tomography showing changes consistent with chronic pancreatitis.

Treatment should primarily be a low-fat diet and abstinence from alcohol. Pancreatic enzyme supplements may reduce steatorrhoea. If conventional medical therapy is unsuccessful and the patient has severe intractable pain, coeliac ganglion blockade can be considered. Surgery is associated with significant morbidity and mortality and relieves symptoms in approximately 75 per cent of patients. It does not result in the return of normal endocrine and exocrine function. Surgery can be performed to bypass an obstructing lesion (pancreaticojejunostomy) or to remove the damaged gland (pancreaticoduodenectomy or distal pancreatectomy).

KEY POINTS

- Thirty per cent of cases of chronic pancreatitis are idiopathic.
- Chronic pancreatitis increases the risk of pancreatic carcinoma.

CASE 33: ABDOMINAL PAIN AND JAUNDICE

History

A general practitioner has referred a 64-year-old woman to the general surgical team on call. She has been complaining of pain in the upper part of the abdomen and generalized itching. Her daughter has also noticed a yellowish discolouration of her skin. The symptoms began about a week ago and have got gradually worse. On further questioning she reports passing dark urine and pale stools for the last few days. She is usually fit and well, does not drink alcohol and denies any recent foreign travel.

Examination

The patient is clinically jaundiced and tender in the right upper abdomen. The liver is not enlarged and rectal examination reveals pale stool on the glove. Her temperature is 37°C, blood pressure 130/80 mmHg and pulse rate 72/min. Bilirubin is detected on urinalysis.

INVESTIGATIONS

		Normal
Haemoglobin	12 g/dL	11.5–16.0 g/dL
Mean cell volume	80 fL	76–96 fL
White cell count	11.5×10^9/L	$4.0–11.0 \times 10^9$/L
Platelets	315×10^9/L	$150–400 \times 10^9$/L
Sodium	137 mmol/L	135–145 mmol/L
Potassium	4.2 mmol/L	3.5–5.0 mmol/L
Urea	6 mmol/L	2.5–6.7 mmmol/L
Creatinine	62 μmol/L	44–80 μmol/L
Amylase	72 IU/dL	0–100 IU/dL
Alkaline phosphatase (ALP)	556 IU/L	35–110 IU/L
Aspartate transaminase (AST)	45 IU/L	5–35 IU/L
Gamma-glutamyl transferase (GGT)	127 IU/L	11–51 IU/L
Albumin	38 g/L	35–50 g/L
Bilirubin	122 mmol/L	3–17 mmol/L

Questions

- What do the blood results show?
- What are the causes of this condition?
- What are the options for investigation and treatment?

ANSWER 33

The patient is jaundiced (bilirubin 122 mmol/L) and the high ALP to AST ratio would suggest the cause is obstructive. The pale stool is because the conjugated bilirubin fails to pass from the liver into the gastrointestinal tract. Conjugated bilirubin is then excreted in the urine giving it a dark appearance. Urinary bilirubin is normally absent and its presence confirms a raised conjugated bilirubin. The causes of obstructive jaundice are shown in Table 33.1.

Table 33.1 Causes of obstructive jaundice

Common	Less frequent	Rare
Common bile duct stones	Ampullary carcinoma	Benign strictures – iatrogenic, trauma
Carcinoma of the head of pancreas	Pancreatitis	Recurrent cholangitis
Malignant porta hepatis lymph nodes	Liver secondaries	Mirrizi's syndrome
		Sclerosing cholangitis
		Cholangiocarcinoma
		Biliary atresia
		Choledochal cysts

Investigation aims to differentiate between hepatocellular and obstructive jaundice. In obstructive jaundice, blood results typically show an elevated conjugated bilirubin (>35 mmol/L) and an increase in ALP/GGT compared to AST/ALT. Ultrasound is the first-line investigation. Gallbladder stones are easily detected (sensitivity >90 per cent), but common bile duct (CBD) stones are frequently missed (sensitivity <40 per cent). The detection of CBD stones can be impeded by the presence of gas in the duodenum. However, CBD dilatation (>8 mm) is identified in up to 90 per cent of cases of CBD obstruction. The liver function tests and the CBD calibre indicate the likelihood of CBD stones.

Based on these findings, patients will either proceed straight to laparoscopic cholecystectomy, or if there is a high risk of a stone(s) in the CBD, an ERCP will be performed to clear the duct prior to surgery. ERCP is used to image the biliary system if therapeutic intervention is likely to be needed. Complications include pancreatitis (less than 1 per cent), perforation, biliary peritonitis, sepsis and haemorrhage. Newer techniques, such as endoscopic ultrasonography and MRCP have a higher sensitivity and specificity of CBD stone detection (85–100 per cent), but are not available in all institutions. These techniques are diagnostic only, but have fewer risks than ERCP. Some surgeons now also advocate intraoperative cholangiography or ultrasonography, negating the need for preoperative imaging in certain cases.

KEY POINTS

- If the bilirubin and ALP are elevated and the CBD is greater than 12 mm, the risk of CBD stones is over 90 per cent.
- If the bilirubin, ALP and CBD diameter are normal, the risk of CBD stones is approximately 0.5 per cent.

CASE 34: POST-PRANDIAL PAIN

History

A 62-year-old man is attending the endoscopy unit for an oesophagogastroscopy. The general practitioner's (GP) letter states that he has been suffering from epigastric pain for the last 6 months. The pain typically occurs about an hour after eating and is associated with nausea and belching. He has had some relief from a proton pump inhibitor, but the symptoms have not entirely settled, despite a 2-month course. Blood tests were arranged by the GP and the results are shown below.

Examination

General examination is normal. A picture taken at endoscopy is shown in Fig. 34.1.

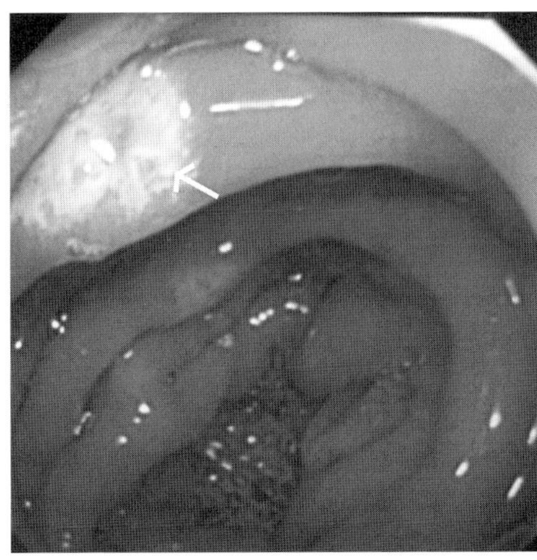

Figure 34.1 Finding on endoscopy.

INVESTIGATIONS

		Normal
Haemoglobin	11.9	11.5–16.0 g/dL
Mean cell volume	86	76–96 fL
White cell count	10	4.0–11.0 × 10^9/L
Platelets	252	150–400 × 10^9/L
Sodium	137	135–145 mmol/L
Potassium	4.2	3.5–5.0 mmol/L
Urea	5.0	2.5–6.7 mmmol/L
Creatinine	72	44–80 μmol/L
Amylase	32	0–100 IU/dL
Aspartate transaminase (AST)	30	5–35 IU/L
Gamma-glutamyl transferase (GGT)	46	11–51 IU/L
Albumin	46	35–50 g/L
Bilirubin	12	3–17 mmol/L
Glucose	5.0	3.5–5.5 mmol/L

Questions

- What is the diagnosis?
- Which common organism is commonly implicated?
- Which other factors are thought to be important?
- Which tests can be used to detect the organism?
- What are the current treatments?

ANSWER 34

Figure 34.1 shows peptic ulceration (arrow). A peptic ulcer is a dissolution in the mucosa, 3 mm or greater in size, of the stomach or duodenum. Epigastric pain is the most common presenting symptom, which often occurs 1–3 h after meals. It can occur at night and is relieved by food or antacids. Nausea is common and vomiting may occur where there is partial or complete gastric outlet obstruction. Patients may also present with haematemesis or melaena resulting from gastrointestinal bleeding. Symptoms do not correlate well with clinical findings, as only 20–25 per cent of patients with symptoms suggestive of peptic ulceration are found to have a peptic ulcer.

Helicobacter pylori is now known to be an important contributory factor in the development of peptic ulceration. It is a gram-negative spiral flagellated bacterium which is found in approximately 90 per cent of patients with duodenal ulceration, 70 per cent of patients with gastric ulceration and 60 per cent of patients with gastric cancer. Normal mucosal production of mucus, bicarbonate and prostaglandins are important in preventing ulceration. A disturbance in this physiological barrier can lead to ulceration. This may be attributed to factors such as smoking, non-steroidal anti-inflammatory drugs (NSAIDs), ethanol, bile acids, aspirin, steroids or stress.

Helicobacter pylori can be detected by biopsies taken at the time of the oesophagogastroduodenoscopy, using a rapid urease test, or by blood serology or a urea breath test. The majority of peptic ulcers will heal after 2 months' treatment with a proton pump inhibitor. There is low recurrence with long-term maintenance therapy. If *Helicobacter pylori is* detected, the patient should have triple therapy, consisting of a 2-week course of amoxicillin, metronidazole and omeprazole.

Patients should be advised to stop smoking, avoid NSAIDs and aspirin use, avoid excessive alcohol and reduce stress.

KEY POINTS

- Most peptic ulcers will heal after 2 months of a high-dose proton pump inhibitor.
- *H. pylori* is found in 90 per cent of patients with duodenal ulceration.

CASE 35: LEFT UPPER QUADRANT MASS

History

The general practitioner (GP) has referred a 63-year-old man to the surgical outpatients. The patient had gone to his GP after becoming lethargic and short of breath on minimal exertion. The GP palpated a mass in the left upper quadrant and noticed multiple bruises on the upper arms and chest. The patient denied any recent injuries.

Examination

On examination, there was no palpable lymphadenopathy, pallor or jaundice. The chest was clear and heart sounds normal. His blood pressure was 136/70 mmHg with a pulse rate of 78/min. Examination of the abdomen revealed a mass in the left upper quadrant. The superior border of the mass could not be reached and a notch was felt on the medial side. The mass was non-pulsatile and dull to percussion. No other masses were palpable and the rest of the examination was unremarkable.

INVESTIGATIONS

		Normal
Haemoglobin	11.2 g/dL	11.5–16.0 g/dL
Mean cell volume	86 fL	76–96 fL
White cell count	4.2×10^9/L	$4.0–11.0 \times 10^9$/L
Platelets	110×10^9/L	$150–400 \times 10^9$/L
Sodium	137 mmol/L	135–145 mmol/L
Potassium	4.2 mmol/L	3.5–5.0 mmol/L
Urea	5 mmol/L	2.5–6.7 mmmol/L
Creatinine	72 μmol/L	44–80 μmol/L
International normalized ratio (INR)	1.0	0.9–1.2
Activated partial thromboplastin time (APTT)	32 s	29–41 s

Examination of the blood film showed teardrop-shaped red blood cells.

Questions

- What is the mass likely to be?
- What are its normal functions?
- What are the causes of enlargement?
- Which condition is this patient likely to have?
- How would the diagnosis be confirmed?
- What are the treatment options?

ANSWER 35

The normal spleen is approximately 11 cm in length and is not normally palpable. The spleen classically enlarges towards the right iliac fossa, has a palpable notch and is dull to percussion. The superior border of the spleen cannot be reached on palpation, differentiating it from renal masses. The spleen is responsible for the synthesis of immunoglobulins and the clearance of micro-organisms, antigens and abnormal red blood cells from the circulation. Enlargement of the spleen is usually due to overactivity of its normal functions.

! Causes of enlargement of the spleen

- *Infective*:
  - *acute*: septicaemia, infective endocarditis, typhoid, infective mononucleosis
  - *chronic*: tuberculosis, hepatitis, brucellosis, HIV
  - *parasitic*: malaria, kala-azar (leishmaniasis), schistosomiasis
- *Inflammatory*:
  - rheumatoid arthritis
  - sarcoidosis
  - systemic lupus erythematosus
- *Haematological*:
  - leukaemia
  - lymphoma
  - haemolysis (thalassaemia, sickle cell disease)
  - myeloproliferative disorders
- *Portal hypertension*
- *Miscellaneous*:
  - storage disorders
  - amyloid
- *Causes of massive splenomegaly*:
  - myelofibrosis
  - chronic myeloid leukaemia
  - chronic malaria
  - kala-azar

The blood film would suggest this patient has myelofibrosis. There is progressive scarring of the bone marrow leading to blood formation in extra-medullary sites, such as the liver and spleen, causing enlargement of these organs. The cause is unknown. The disorder usually develops slowly, in people over 50 years of age. It leads to progressive bone-marrow failure with severe anaemia. The diagnosis is made on examination of the blood films, showing teardrop-shaped red blood cells, and on bone-marrow biopsy.

There is no specific treatment for primary myelofibrosis. Blood transfusions and erythropoietin are given to correct the anaemia. A splenectomy may help if the enlarged size of the spleen causes thrombocytopenia. Splenectomy can be performed through a subcostal incision or laparoscopically. The patient should be cross-matched prior to the procedure, and platelets ordered if the platelet count is low. Those patients who undergo splenectomy, have a lifetime risk of septicaemia and should receive immunizations against *Pneumococcus*, *Haemophilus* and *Meningococcus*.

KEY POINTS

The characteristics of the spleen on clinical examination are:

- the superior border cannot be felt
- the medial border is notched
- it is dull to percussion
- it enlarges towards the right iliac fossa.

CASE 36: FINDING AT GASTROSCOPY

History

A general practitioner (GP) has referred a 56-year-old man for an oesophagogastroduodenoscopy. The patient presented to the GP 2 months previously with epigastric discomfort and bloating. He was prescribed a proton pump inhibitor which failed to improve his symptoms. He has no history of gastro-oesophageal reflux or gallstones and is not on any other regular medication. He smokes 20 cigarettes a day. The GP also sent some blood tests shown below.

INVESTIGATIONS

		Normal
Haemoglobin	9.0 g/dL	11.5–16.0 g/dL
Mean cell volume	69 fL	76–96 fL
White cell count	10.2 × 10^9/L	4.0–11.0 × 10^9/L
Platelets	252 × 10^9/L	150–400 × 10^9/L
Sodium	137 mmol/L	135–145 mmol/L
Potassium	3.9 mmol/L	3.5–5.0 mmol/L
Urea	5.0 mmol/L	2.5–6.7 mmmol/L
Creatinine	59 μmol/L	44–80 μmol/L
Amylase	78 IU/dL	0–100 IU/dL
Aspartate transaminase (AST)	30 IU/dL	5–35 IU/L
Gamma-glutamyl transferase (GGT)	23 IU/dL	11–51 IU/L
Albumin	45 g/L	35–50 g/L
Bilirubin	12 mmol/L	3–17 mmol/L
Glucose	5.0 mmol/L	3.5–5.5 mmol/L

The endoscopy results are shown in Fig. 36.1.

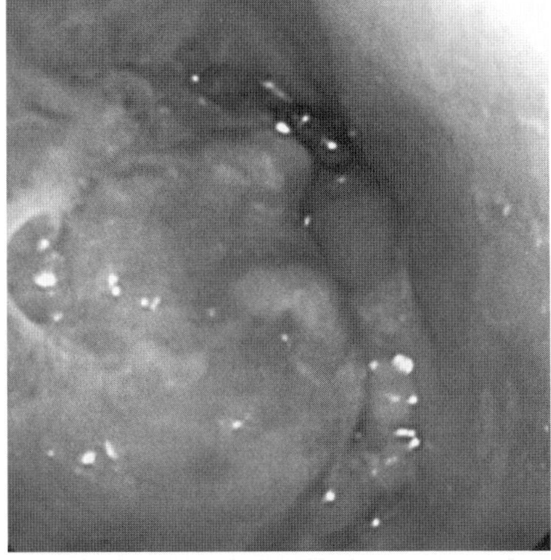

Figure 36.1 Finding on endoscopy.

Questions

- What does the endoscopy show?
- What do the blood tests reveal?
- What are the risk factors for this diagnosis?
- How should the patient be staged?
- What are the treatment options?

ANSWER 36

The gastroscopy has revealed a gastric tumour. The blood tests show a microcytic anaemia, as a result of chronic blood loss from the tumour. This patient will have had multiple biopsies taken at endoscopy and will now require staging. Gastric carcinoma is the second commonest cause of cancer worldwide. The majority are adenocarcinomas with the remainder made up of lymphomas, stromal or neuroendocrine tumours. The highest incidence is in Eastern Asia, with a falling incidence in Western Europe. Diet and *Helicobacter pylori* infection are thought to be the two most important environmental factors in the development of gastric cancer. Diets rich in pickled vegetables, salted fish and smoked meats are thought to predispose to gastric cancer. These factors contribute to a premature atrophic gastritis, a precursor state to malignant transformation. Fruits and vegetables are protective.

! Risk factors for gastric malignancy

- Vitamin C deficiency
- *H. pylori* infection
- Hypogammaglobulinaemia
- Pernicious anaemia
- Post-gastrectomy

Gastric cancer typically presents late and is associated with a poor prognosis. Clinical examination may reveal supraclavicular lymphadenopathy or hepatic enlargement, indicative of metastatic disease. Endoscopic ultrasound allows assessment of tumour depth and nodal involvement. Computerized tomography also allows nodal spread and the extent of metastatic disease to be assessed (Fig. 36.2).

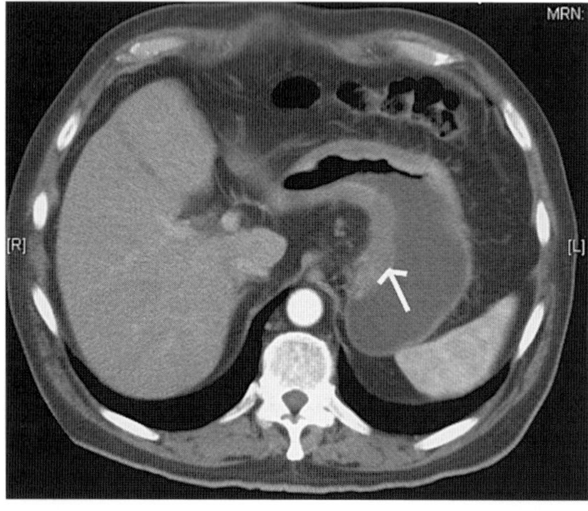

Figure 36.2 Computerized tomography showing gastric wall thickening (arrow) as a result of gastric cancer. No liver metastases are seen.

Laparoscopy is useful to identify any peritoneal seedlings that are not detected on conventional imaging.

Antral tumours may be suitable for a partial gastrectomy. If the tumour is less than 5 cm from the gastro-esophageal junction, the patient will require a total gastrectomy. For tumours less than 1 cm in size, some centres are now carrying out endoscopic mucosal resection. If the tumour extends into the submucosa the patient is unsuitable for this technique.

Results from adjuvant chemotherapy are disappointing, with only small improvements in survival after surgical resection. Neoadjuvant chemotherapy is still under assessment.

KEY POINTS

- Gastric cancer often presents late with metastatic disease.
- Surgical resection is not possible in the majority of patients.

BREAST AND ENDOCRINE

CASE 37: ASSESSMENT OF A BREAST LUMP

History

A 47-year-old female presents to the breast clinic complaining of a painful lump in her left breast. She has not noticed any nipple discharge, skin changes or changes in her breast shape. Her mother was diagnosed with breast cancer at 50 years of age. She has recently been through a divorce and has no children. She is a non-smoker and has been previously fit and healthy.

Examination

A 4 cm irregular lump is found adjacent to the nipple in the left breast. The lump is hard in consistency and only mildly tender on palpation. It is slightly mobile with no tethering of the overlying skin. It does not appear deeply fixed. There are palpable left-sided axillary lymph nodes which are mobile. The right breast and axilla are normal. Abdominal and skeletal examinations are normal.

INVESTIGATIONS

A mammogram of the breast is shown in Fig. 37.1.

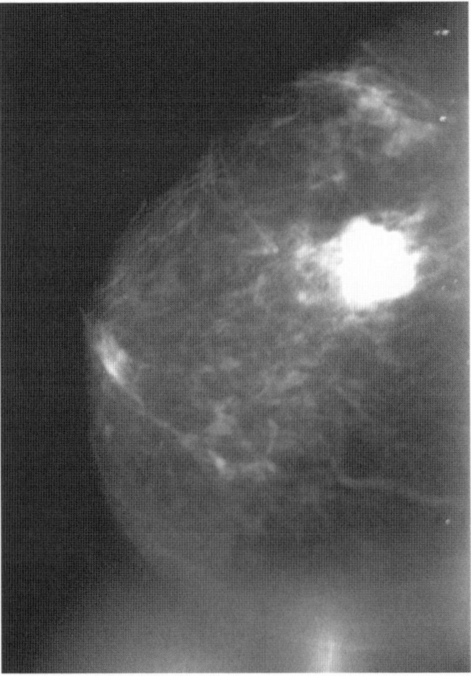

Figure 37.1 Mammogram of the left breast.

Questions

- How should this lump be assessed?
- What are the risk factors for developing breast cancer?
- To what age group does the UK offer a breast screening programme?
- What is a sentinel lymph node biopsy?

ANSWER 37

Breast cancer is the commonest form of cancer amongst women. Any women presenting with a breast lump should undergo triple assessment:

- clinical assessment (history/examination)
- mammography and/or ultrasound
- fine-needle aspiration cytology (FNAC) or core biopsy.

The incidence increases with age, but at menopause the rate of increase slows. Risk factors for developing breast cancer include:

- oestrogen exposure, unopposed by progesterone
- nulliparous women in developed countries
- mutations in the *BRCA1* and *BRCA2* genes
- early menarche/late menopause
- family history
- saturated dietary fats
- previous benign atypical hyperplasia.

The breast screening programme was set up by the Department of Health in 1988 and is offered to women between the ages of 50 and 70 years. All women now have two views of the breast taken at every screen – craniocaudal and mediolateral views. It has reduced mortality rates in the 55–69-year age group.

In patients without systemic disease, surgery is potentially curative. Treatment options include mastectomy or breast-conservation surgery, such as wide local excision or quadrantectomy. Axillary lymph node status is a good prognostic indicator for breast cancer and is helpful in delineating further treatment pathways. Management of the axilla is controversial. Options include axillary node sampling, clearance or sentinel node biopsy. The sentinel node is the first lymph node the breast lymphatics drain to before reaching the axilla. Sentinel lymph node biopsy is an alternative to axillary sampling or clearance which provides information on the probable tumour status of other axillary lymph nodes. The technique involves injection of a technetium-based radioisotope into the breast, often in combination with a dye. The sentinel node is detected with the use of a gamma camera or direct visualization on dissection (the dye is usually blue) before excision.

KEY POINT

- All patients presenting with a lump in the breast should undergo triple assessment.

CASE 38: BREAST LUMP ON SELF-EXAMINATION

History

A 33-year-old woman is referred to the breast clinic after noticing a painless lump in her right breast during self-examination. She reports no associated nipple discharge or skin changes and is currently mid-menstrual cycle. She has a 3-year-old daughter and has no family history of breast disease. She smokes 15 cigarettes per day.

Examination

On examination of the right breast, a 3 cm lump is found in the upper outer quadrant. It is rubbery in consistency, mobile and non-tender. There are no skin changes. There is no evidence of lymphadenopathy in either axillae or supraclavicular fossae. The left breast is normal and abdominal examination is unremarkable.

Questions

- What are the possible diagnoses?
- What is the likely diagnosis in this patient?
- How should this be confirmed?
- How should the patient be managed?

ANSWER 38

The most likely diagnosis is a benign fibroadenoma. They are most commonly seen between the ages of 15 and 35 years. The fibromatous element is the dominant feature. They tend to grow slowly and occasionally can grow to >5 cm, where they are termed giant fibroadenomata. Fibroadenomata are often multiple and bilateral and are often referred to as 'breast mice' because they are extremely mobile. On examination they tend to be spherical, smooth and sometimes lobulated with a rubbery consistency. The differential diagnosis includes fibrocystic disease (fluctuation in size with menstrual cycle and often associated with mild tenderness), a breast cyst (smooth, well-defined consistency like fibroadenoma but a hard as opposed to a rubbery consistency) or breast carcinoma (irregular, indistinct surface and shape with hard consistency).

Confirmation of the diagnosis should be with fine-needle aspiration cytology (FNAC) or excision biopsy. If FNAC is performed, treatment options include wide local excision or observation, depending on patient wishes. Malignant change occurs in 1 in 1000.

KEY POINT

- A diagnosis of benign fibroadenoma should be confirmed by triple assessment.

CASE 39: BREAST INFECTION

History

A 26-year-old woman who is 5 weeks post partum presents with right breast pain and a fever. She is breast-feeding her son. Over the last 3 weeks she has seen her general practitioner (GP) on two occasions with mastitis and has been prescribed antibiotics. However, the pain is now worsening and she is starting to feel more unwell. She is normally fit and healthy. She does not take any regular medications and is allergic to penicillin.

Examination

She has a temperature of 37.9°C and a pulse rate of 92/min. On examination, there is a localized, tender area, adjacent to the areola of the right breast. There is surrounding erythema and tender lymphadenopathy in the right axilla.

INVESTIGATIONS

		Normal
Haemoglobin	11.3 g/dL	11.5–16.0 g/dL
Mean cell volume	86 fL	76–96 fL
White cell count	16.8×10^9/L	$4.0–11.0 \times 10^9$/L
Neutrophils	12.8×10^9/L	$1.7–6.1 \times 10^9$/L
Platelets	345×10^9	$150–400 \times 10^9$/L

Questions

- What is the likely diagnosis?
- What other investigations would you arrange?
- What are the treatment options, and what other considerations do you have to make when prescribing?
- What other advice would you give regarding her breast-feeding?

ANSWER 39

This woman has a puerperal breast abscess. Mastitis occurs frequently in lactating females. Infection is most common in the first 6 weeks post partum. This is the result of organisms entering through traumatized skin and cracked nipples. It is usually treated with antibiotics, and mothers are advised to continue expressing from the breast to aid drainage through the ducts. Occasionally the infection can progress and lead to a breast abscess. The most commonly involved organisms are *Staphylococcus aureus* and the *Streptococcus* species.

Non-lactating breast abscesses occur most commonly around the age of 30 years and are often associated with duct ectasia. Periareolar abscesses are found to be associated with smoking, whereas peripheral abscesses are more common in immunosuppressed women, such as those taking steroids or patients with diabetes.

In this case other investigations would include anaerobic and aerobic cultures taken from the abscess. These can usually be obtained by needle aspiration under ultrasound guidance.

Treatment is either by recurrent needle aspiration or by incision and drainage. Antibiotics should be continued. Flucloxacillin (or erythromycin if the patient is penicillin allergic) are recommended, but the choice of antibiotic should be guided by the culture results. Co-amoxiclav is prescribed in non-lactating breast abscesses where anaerobes and enterococci may also be causative. Appropriate analgesia should also be prescribed. It is imperative to remember that this patient is breast-feeding and the *British National Formulary* (*BNF* – Appendix 4) should be consulted before prescribing to ensure there are no contraindications.

KEY POINT

- It is important to note that if the inflammation or mass persists after treatment, then the possibility of breast cancer should be ruled out with further imaging and tissue sampling.

CASE 40: SWELLING IN THE NECK

History

A 45-year-old woman is referred to the general surgical outpatients after her general practitioner (GP) noticed a swelling in the neck. On questioning, the patient reports losing about a stone in weight over the preceding 3 months, despite having an increased appetite. She also complains that she always feels hot and has to sleep on top of the bed covers at night. Her bowel motions have been loose.

Examination

The patient is thin, irritable and has a noticeable fine resting tremor. Her peripheries feel warm and she has a resting heart rate of 110/min, with a blood pressure of 150/90 mmHg. On examination of the neck, there is a smooth moderate enlargement of the thyroid gland, which moves on swallowing. There is protrusion of the eyes with lid retraction. Her visual acuity and eye movements are normal. There is no associated lymphadenopathy. The heart sounds are normal and the chest is clear.

INVESTIGATIONS

		Normal
Haemoglobin	12.0 g/dL	11.5–16.0 g/dL
Mean cell volume	77 fL	76–96 fL
White cell count	10.4×10^9/L	$4.0–11.0 \times 10^9$/L
Platelets	250×10^9/L	$150–400 \times 10^9$/L
Sodium	137 mmol/L	135–145 mmol/L
Potassium	3.7 mmol/L	3.5–5.0 mmol/L
Urea	5 mmol/L	2.5–6.7 mmmol/L
Creatinine	79 μmol/L	44–80 μmol/L
Thyroid-stimulating hormone (TSH)	0.01 mu/L	0.5–5.7 mu/L
Tri-iodothyronine (T_3)	17 pmol/L	2.5–5.3 pmol/L
Thyroxine (T_4)	42 pmol/L	9–22 pmol/L

Questions

- What are the causes of a goitre?
- What is the likely diagnosis in this patient?
- What are the options for treatment?

ANSWER 40

A goitre is an enlargement of the thyroid gland. It can be diffuse or multinodular in origin.

! Causes of goitre

- *Diffuse*:
  - physiological: puberty/pregnancy
  - autoimmune: Graves' disease/Hashimoto's thyroiditis
  - inflammatory: De Quervain's (acute) thyroiditis/Riedel's (chronic) thyroiditis
  - iodine deficiency: colloid/simple
  - goitrogens: carbimazole/propylthiouracil
  - lymphoma
- *Multinodular/solitary nodule*:
  - multinodular goitre
  - cysts
  - tumours: adenomas/carcinoma
  - miscellaneous: sarcoidosis/tuberculosis

This patient has hyperthyroidism secondary to Graves' disease. The TSH levels are suppressed and there are increased levels of free T_3 and T_4. Graves' disease most commonly develops in women aged between 30 and 50 years and is caused by circulating stimulating antibodies to the thyroid receptors (LATS). Patients often present with many symptoms including palpitations, anxiety, thirst, sweating, weight loss, heat intolerance and increased bowel frequency. Enhanced activity of the adrenergic system also leads to agitation and restlessness. Approximately 25–30 per cent of patients with Graves' disease have clinical evidence of ophthalmopathy. This almost only occurs in Graves' disease (very rarely found in hypothyroidism) and is also due to autoantibody damage leading to swelling of the orbital fat and connective tissue. Low titres of microsomal and thyroglobulin antibodies are also often present in patients with Graves' disease.

Many patients are now treated with radio-iodine therapy. Antithyroid medication, carbimazole or propylthiouracil, are used to establish control of hyperthyroidism and act by inhibiting thyroid hormone production. Beta-blockers may also be used initially to control symptoms. Surgery is indicated in patients with a large goitre, in patients with recurring disease and in patients unable to have radio-iodine therapy (patients planning pregnancy). There is a surgical risk of damage to the recurrent laryngeal nerve (1 per cent), hypocalcaemia (1 per cent) and hypothyroidism (10 per cent).

KEY POINTS

- Graves' disease is caused by antibodies to the thyroid receptors.
- Up to 30 per cent of patients with Graves' disease have eye signs.

CASE 41: A PAINLESS LUMP IN THE NECK

History

A 40-year-old woman has been referred to the surgical outpatients with a painless lump in the neck. She had noticed the lump 2 weeks previously when looking in the mirror. She had not noticed any other lumps and does not complain of any other symptoms. She has not gained or lost any weight recently and her bowel habit has remained normal.

Examination

Examination reveals a solitary 2 × 2 cm swelling to the left of the midline just above the manubrium. The swelling is firm, smooth and fixed. The swelling moves on swallowing, but does not move on protrusion of the tongue. There are no associated palpable lymph glands. General examination reveals no further abnormalities.

INVESTIGATIONS

		Normal
Haemoglobin	12.0 g/dL	11.5–16.0 g/dL
Mean cell volume	77 fL	76–96 fL
White cell count	10.4×10^9/L	$4.0–11.0 \times 10^9$/L
Platelets	250×10^9/L	$150–400 \times 10^9$/L
Sodium	137 mmol/L	135–145 mmol/L
Potassium	3.7 mmol/L	3.5–5.0 mmol/L
Urea	5 mmol/L	2.5–6.7 mmmol/L
Creatinine	71 μmol/L	44–80 μmol/L
Thyroid-stimulating hormone (TSH)	0.62 mu/L	0.5–5.7 mu/L
Free tri-iodothyronine (T_3)	3.4 pmol/L	2.5–5.3 pmol/L
Free thyroxine (T_4)	19 pmol/L	9–22 pmol/L

Questions

- What is the differential diagnosis for a lump in the anterior triangle of the neck?
- Where is this lump likely to be originating from?
- What steps would you take in the assessment of this lump?
- Which factors may suggest malignancy?
- What are the commonest types of malignancy?

ANSWER 41

! Differentials for a swelling in the anterior triangle of the neck

- *Multiple*: lymph nodes
- *Solitary*: does it move with swallowing?
  - *yes*:
    - thyroid origin
    - thyroglossal cyst (moves with protrusion of the tongue)
  - *no*:
    - salivary gland
    - dermoid cyst
    - carotid body tumour
    - lymph node
    - branchial cyst
    - cold abscess (TB)

Clinical examination indicates that the swelling is likely to be a palpable thyroid nodule. The majority of patients are clinically euthyroid and have normal thyroid function. The presence of abnormal thyroid function suggests a benign diagnosis. Factors that increase the suspicion of malignancy include:

- age younger than 20 years or older than 70 years
- male sex
- recent origin and rapid growth or increase in size
- firm, hard, or immobile nodule
- presence of cervical lymphadenopathy
- associated symptoms of dysphagia or dysphonia
- history of neck irradiation
- prior history of thyroid carcinoma or a positive family history.

Less than 20 per cent of thyroid nodules are malignant, with the majority being cystic or benign. Many solitary thyroid nodules are dominant nodules in a multinodular goitre, which carry a 5 per cent risk of malignancy. Ultrasound is used to distinguish between solid and cystic nodules as well as differentiating a solitary nodule from a dominant nodule in a multinodular goitre. Fine-needle aspiration has a high sensitivity and specificity for distinguishing benign from malignant lumps in the thyroid. The main limitation of fine-needle aspiration is in the differentiation of benign follicular adenoma from malignant follicular cancer. If a follicular neoplasm is diagnosed on fine-needle aspiration, the lesion will need to be fully excised to exclude malignancy. Radio-isotope scanning provides a functional assessment of the thyroid nodule, which can be classified as cold or hot. Most solitary thyroid nodules are cold, with a risk of cancer at around 20 per cent.

Table 41.1 Types of thyroid cancer

Type	Frequency	Age (years)	Behaviour	Prognosis
Papillary	70%	20–40s	Slow growing, lymphatic spread to nodes	Good, ~80% 10-year survival
Follicular	20%	35–50s	Bloodstream spread, metastasizes to lung or bone	Good, ~60% 10-year survival
Anaplastic	<5%	60–70s	Aggressive, local spread	Poor, ~10% 10-year survival
Medullary	5%	Familial	From parafollicular C cells, associated with the multiple endocrine neoplasia (MEN) syndrome	

 **KEY POINTS**

- Less than 20 per cent of thyroid nodules are malignant.
- Follicular adenomas should be excised to rule out malignancy.

VASCULAR

CASE 42: A PULSATILE MASS IN THE ABDOMEN

History

A 68-year-old man presents to the emergency department with a 1 h history of pain in the left side of his abdomen. The pain started suddenly while he was getting up from a chair. It became constant and radiated through to his back. His past medical history includes hypertension and stable angina. He lives with his wife and is normally independent.

Examination

The patient is pale, sweaty and clammy. His pulse is 100/min and the blood pressure is 90/50 mmHg. Heart sounds are normal and the chest is clear. Examination of the abdomen reveals a large tender mass in the epigastrium. The mass is both pulsatile and expansile. The peripheral pulses are present and equal on both sides. There is no neurological deficit.

INVESTIGATIONS

		Normal
Haemoglobin	9.3 g/dL	11.5–16.0 g/dL
Mean cell volume	86 fL	76–96 fL
White cell count	5×10^9/L	$4.0–11.0 \times 10^9$/L
Platelets	250×10^9/L	$150–400 \times 10^9$/L
Sodium	143 mmol/L	135–145 mmol/L
Potassium	4.4 mmol/L	3.5–5.0 mmol/L
Urea	4.2 mmol/L	2.5–6.7 mmmol/L
Creatinine	72 μmol/L	44–80 μmol/L
C-reactive protein	20 mg/L	<5 mg/L
Amylase	22 IU/dL	0–100 IU/dL

Questions

- What is the most likely diagnosis?
- What is required in the immediate management of this patient?
- What is the prognosis?

ANSWER 42

The most likely diagnosis is a ruptured abdominal aortic aneurysm. An aortic aneurysm is defined as an increase in aortic diameter by greater than 50 per cent of normal (>3 cm). The aneurysm diameter increases exponentially by approximately 10 per cent per year. As the aneurysm expands, so does the risk of rupture:

Aneurysm size:

- 5.0–5.9 cm, ~25 per cent 5-year risk of rupture
- 6.0–6.9 cm, ~35 per cent 5-year risk of rupture
- more than 7 cm, ~75 per cent 5-year risk of rupture.

Aneurysm rupture (Fig. 42.1) can present with abdominal pain radiating to the back, groin or iliac fossae. An expansile mass is not always detectable and other conditions, such as acute pancreatitis or mesenteric infarction, should always be considered. Intravenous access should be established quickly with two large-bore cannulae. Ten units of cross-matched blood, fresh-frozen plasma and platelets should be requested. The bladder should be catheterized and an electrocardiogram (ECG) obtained. It is important not to resuscitate the patient aggressively as a high blood pressure may cause a second fatal bleed. The patient should be taken immediately to theatre and prepared for surgery. A vascular clamp is placed onto the aorta above the leak and a graft used to replace the aneurysmal segment. Some centres now practise endovascular stenting of ruptured aneurysms in a patient stable enough to undergo computerized tomography (CT) scanning.

The mortality from a ruptured aneurysm is high, with haemorrhage, multi-organ failure, myocardial infarction and cerebrovascular accidents accounting for most deaths.

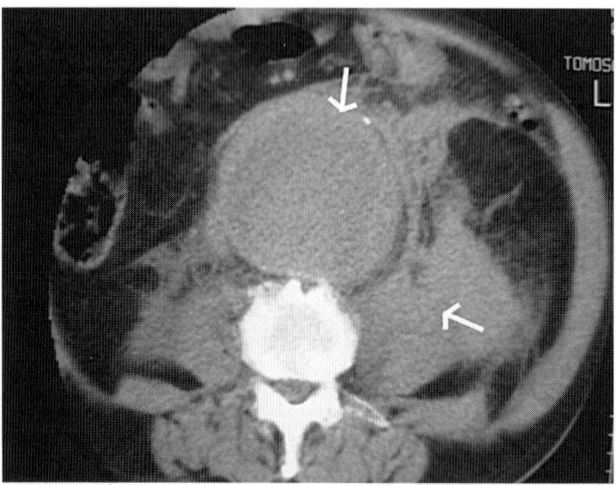

Figure 42.1 Abdominal computerized tomography scan demonstrating a ruptured abdominal aortic aneurysm (top arrow) and retroperitoneal haematoma (lower arrow).

KEY POINTS

- Aneurysms less than 5.5 cm in diameter should be monitored.
- Aneurysms greater than 5.5 cm in diameter should be considered for surgical intervention.

CASE 43: HEADACHE, LETHARGY AND BLURRED VISION

History

A 76-year-old man presents to his general practitioner (GP) with a 2-day history of headache and blurred vision. He describes general lethargy and muscle aching over the last 3–4 days. On further questioning, he reports that when brushing his hair he experiences pain on the same side of his forehead as the headache. His GP has recently started a statin for raised cholesterol and he takes bendroflumethiazide 2.5 mg once daily for hypertension.

Examination

His general examination is unremarkable, blood pressure 136/86 mmHg and pulse 78/min.

INVESTIGATIONS

		Normal
Haemoglobin	13.2 g/dL	11.5–16.0 g/dL
Mean cell volume	86 fL	76–96 fL
White cell count	9×10^9/L	$4.0–11.0 \times 10^9$/L
Platelets	355×10^9/L	$150–400 \times 10^9$/L
Erythrocyte sedimentation rate (ESR)	100 mm/h	10–20 mm/h
Sodium	132 mmol/L	135–145 mmol/L
Potassium	3.9 mmol/L	3.5–5.0 mmol/L
Urea	5.1 mmol/L	2.5–6.7 mmmol/L
Creatinine	69 μmol/L	44–80 μmol/L
Glucose	6 mmol/L	3.5–5.5 mmol/L

Questions

- What is the likely diagnosis?
- What should the initial management involve?

ANSWER 43

The most likely diagnosis is temporal arteritis. This condition predominantly affects the elderly population. Temporal arteritis is usually a clinical diagnosis, which is suggested by its unilateral features (bilateral presentation is rare), typically of pain affecting the temporal region, and can be associated visual disturbance. Palpation of the affected artery may reveal tenderness, warmth, and pulselessness. The inflamed artery may be dilated and thickened, allowing the vessel to be rolled between the fingers and skull. Jaw claudication may occur when the patient is chewing or talking and is seen in approximately 65 per cent of patients with temporal arteritis. Constitutional symptoms include anorexia, weight loss, fever, sweats and malaise. The ESR is characteristically over 100 mm/h.

The importance of making the diagnosis is that without high-dose oral steroids the patient can permanently lose vision on the affected side. Oral steroid treatment usually results in an improvement in symptoms within 48 h, and such a response further supports the diagnosis. The length of the treatment course is 12–18 months.

To confirm the diagnosis, a temporal artery biopsy can be performed. This should ideally be performed within 2 weeks of commencing treatment. It is important to note that a negative biopsy does not rule out the presence of temporal arteritis as the areas of inflammation affecting the temporal artery may not be uniform and can skip regions.

KEY POINT

- The importance of making the diagnosis is that without high-dose oral steroids the patient can permanently lose vision on the affected side.

CASE 44: TRANSIENT ARM WEAKNESS

History

A 71-year-old man presents to the emergency department with weakness and numbness in his left arm. The symptoms came on suddenly while he was in the garden 2 h ago. His vision was not affected and he thinks the weakness in his arm has now resolved. He has had no previous episodes and has no history of trauma to his head or neck. He is currently on medication for hypertension and is a lifelong smoker.

Examination

The blood pressure is 130/90 mmHg and the pulse rate is regular at 90/min. Heart sounds are normal and the chest is clear. Abdominal examination is normal. Neurological examination does not show any neurological deficit. A right-sided carotid bruit is heard.

Questions

- What is the diagnosis?
- What are the risk factors?
- How should this patient be investigated?
- What are the complications of surgery?

ANSWER 44

A transient ischaemic attack (TIA) refers to a focal neurological deficit which lasts less than 24 h. A stroke is a deficit lasting more than 24 h. Eighty per cent of cerebrovascular incidents are caused by emboli, with the majority of infarctions in the carotid territory.

! Risk factors

- Hypertension
- Smoking
- Diabetes mellitus
- Atrial fibrillation
- Raised cholesterol

Patients should undergo the following investigations:

- full blood count, erythrocyte sedimentation rate
- electrocardiogram
- imaging of the carotid, which can be done by:
  - duplex ultrasonography: this technique combines B mode ultrasound and colour Doppler flow to assess the site and degree of stenosis. This is now the investigation of choice in most centres
  - angiography: intra-arterial angiography is the gold standard but is invasive and is associated with a 1–2 per cent risk of stroke. Intravenous digital subtraction angiography is used in some centres
  - magnetic resonance angiography
  - spiral computerized tomography (CT) angiography
- CT head scan: to delineate areas of infarction and exclude haemorrhage in an acute presentation with stroke.

A stenosis of more than 70 per cent in the internal carotid artery is an indication for carotid endarterectomy in a patient with TIAs (Fig. 44.1).

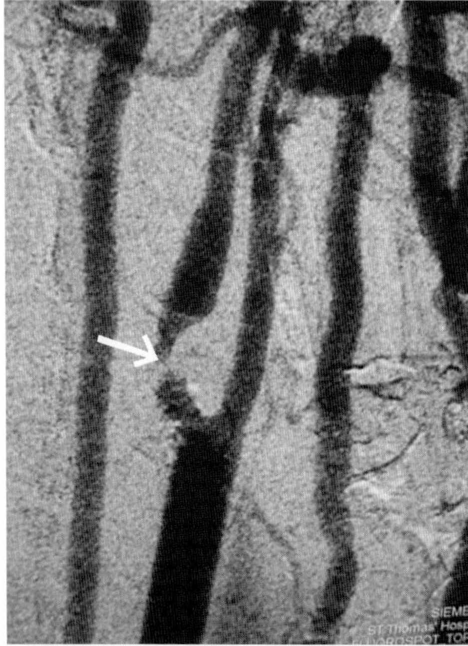

Figure 44.1 Internal carotid artery stenosis (arrow) on angiography.

Risks of surgery

- Neck haematoma (5 per cent)
- Cervical and cranial nerve injury (7 per cent): hypoglossal, vagus, recurrent laryngeal, marginal mandibular and transverse cervical nerves
- Stroke (2 per cent)
- Myocardial infarction
- False aneurysm: rare
- Infection of prosthetic patch: rare
- Death (1 per cent)

KEY POINTS

- Symptoms in a transient ischaemic attack last less than 24 h.
- Symptomatic carotid stenosis of >70 per cent should be considered for carotid endarterectomy.

CASE 45: ABDOMINAL PAIN AND METABOLIC ACIDOSIS

History

A 65-year-old man presents to the emergency department with an 8 h history of severe generalized abdominal pain. Earlier in the day he passed fresh blood mixed in with his stool. His past medical history includes diabetes, hypertension and atrial fibrillation. He is not currently taking any anticoagulation therapy for his atrial fibrillation. He smokes 20 cigarettes per day.

Examination

He has difficulty lying still on the bed. He has a temperature of 37.5°C with an irregularly irregular pulse of 110/min. His blood pressure is 90/50 mmHg. Abdominal examination shows generalized tenderness with absent bowel sounds. Rectal examination confirms loose stool mixed with some fresh blood.

INVESTIGATIONS

		Normal
Haemoglobin	12.2 g/dL	11.5–16.0 g/dL
Mean cell volume	86 fL	76–96 fL
White cell count	13.2 $\times 10^9$/L	4.0–11.0 $\times 10^9$/L
Platelets	252 $\times 10^9$/L	150–400 $\times 10^9$/L
Sodium	138 mmol/L	135–145 mmol/L
Potassium	4.4 mmol/L	3.5–5.0 mmol/L
Urea	3.2 mmol/L	2.5–6.7 mmmol/L
Creatinine	72 μmol/L	44–80 μmol/L
C-reactive protein	36 mg/L	<5 mg/L
Amylase	126 IU/dL	0–100 IU/dl
pH	7.29	7.36–7.44
Partial pressure of CO_2 (pCO_2)	3.5 kPa	4.7–5.9 kPa
Partial pressure of O_2 (pO_2)	8.9 kPa	11–13 kPa
Base excess	–6.5	±2
Lactate	9.4	<2 mmol/L

Questions

- What does the arterial blood gas show?
- What is the most likely diagnosis?
- What are the differential diagnoses?
- What other investigations can you suggest?
- What is the treatment and prognosis for this condition?

ANSWER 45

The arterial blood gas shows a metabolic acidosis (low pH, negative base excess and high lactate) with partial respiratory compensation (low pco_2). The most likely diagnosis is mesenteric ischaemia secondary to superior mesenteric artery thrombosis or embolism. Atrial fibrillation is a risk factor for embolism.

Differential diagnoses

- Pancreatitis
- Ruptured abdominal aortic aneurysm
- Perforated viscus

Investigation should include:

- routine bloods and serum amylase to exclude pancreatitis
- electrocardiogram
- chest X-ray: may show free air under the diaphragm
- abdominal X-ray: typically 'gasless'
- computerized tomography of the abdomen: not always diagnostic with ischaemic bowel but would help to exclude an abdominal aortic aneurysm.

The prognosis associated with this condition is poor, with less than 20 per cent survival. The patient should be resuscitated with intravenous fluids and broad-spectrum antibiotics given. The patient should then be taken for urgent laparotomy where any dead bowel is resected. Revascularization by embolectomy or bypass may improve doubtfully viable bowel and allow primary anastamosis. Otherwise, both ends of the bowel should be exteriorized.

KEY POINTS

- Atrial fibrillation increases the risk of arterial embolization.
- A re-look laparotomy at 24 h may be required to check for further intestinal ischaemia.

CASE 46: PAINFUL FINGERS

History

A 30-year-old woman attends the surgical outpatient clinic complaining of painful fingers. She notices the pain particularly during the winter months when it is colder. When she is outside, the fingers firstly become white, then blue and then become red and start to tingle. She smokes ten cigarettes per day and is currently taking atenolol for hypertension.

Examination

On examination the fingers have a reddish tinge and the skin feels dry. Examination of the neck is normal and all pulses in the upper limbs are present.

Questions

- What is the most likely diagnosis?
- Can you explain the sequence of colour changes?
- What are the environmental factors that can exacerbate this condition?
- What investigations would you carry out?
- What treatments would you suggest?

ANSWER 46

This is Raynaud's phenomenon. When this disorder occurs without any known cause, it is called Raynaud's disease, or primary Raynaud's. When the condition has a likely cause, it is known as Raynaud's phenomenon.

The majority of patients are female (up to 90 per cent) and the prevalence of this condition can be as high as 20 per cent in the general population. Raynaud's can affect the hands, feet and even the tip of the nose. Digital artery spasm results in blanching of the fingers; the accumulation of de-oxygenated blood then gives the fingers a bluish tinge and finally the fingers become red due to reactive hyperaemia. Accumulation of metabolites causes paraesthesia.

! Causes of Raynaud's phenomenon

- Systemic lupus erythematosus
- Systemic sclerosis (scleroderma)
- Rheumatoid arthritis
- Cold agglutinins
- Polycythaemia
- Oral contraceptives
- Beta-blockers such as atenolol (as in this case)
- Occupational (vibrating tools)
- Cervical rib

Tests to rule out a possible cause include a full blood count, urea and electrolytes, cryoglobulins, erythrocyte sedimentation rate, rheumatoid antibodies, antinuclear factor and anti-mitochondrial antibodies. Duplex scanning can be used to assess the arterial supply of the limb.

It is important to keep the extremities warm and avoid the cold by use of gloves/warm socks or even moving to a warmer climate if possible. Drugs (e.g. beta-blockers, contraceptives) that exacerbate the condition should be stopped. Similarly smokers should be encouraged to stop. Calcium-blocking drugs (e.g. nifedipine) and 5-hydroxytryptamine antagonists have all been used with some success.

KEY POINT

- Medications should be excluded as a cause of Raynaud's phenomenon.

CASE 47: DIABETIC FOOT

History

A 54-year-old insulin-dependent diabetic woman has come to the emergency department complaining of increasing pain in the right foot for the past week. The pain is worse at night and is relieved by hanging her leg over the side of the bed. For the last few days she has noticed swelling, redness and discolouration over the base of the big toe. Her glucose control has been recently reviewed by the general practice nurse and her insulin regimen changed.

Examination

She is afebrile, her pulse is 86/min, her blood pressure is 130/60 mmHg and her blood glucose is 13.2 mmol/L on BM stick testing. Femoral pulses are palpable bilaterally. No popliteal, posterior tibial or dorsalis pedis pulses are palpable in either limb. The great toe is erythematous with a large fluctuant swelling at the base.

INVESTIGATIONS

An X-ray of the foot is shown in Fig. 47.1.

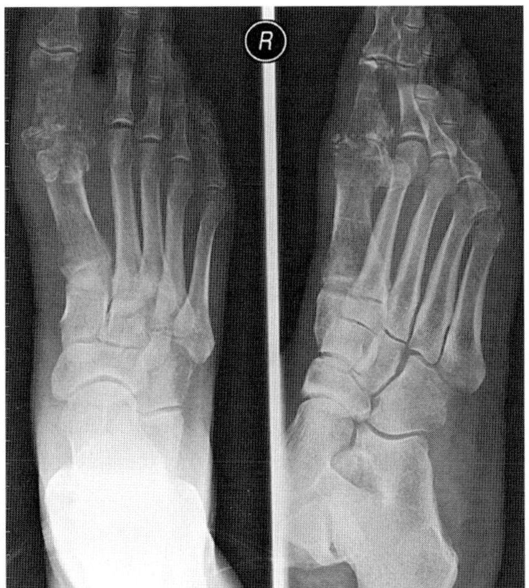

Figure 47.1 Plain X-ray of the foot.

Questions

- What do the clinical appearances suggest?
- What does the X-ray show?
- What other investigations does she require?
- How would you manage this patient?

ANSWER 47

This patient has peripheral vascular disease and poor diabetic control. Examination describes swelling and erythema over the base of the first metatarsal, which may indicate an underlying collection of pus. A full vascular examination should be carried out and ankle–brachial indices measured. All areas of the foot, especially between the toes and the heel should be examined for other areas of ulceration, and the foot examined for the presence of diabetic neuropathy.

Investigations should include:

- full blood count
- renal function and C-reactive protein
- blood sugar
- foot X-ray.

The patient should be commenced on intravenous broad-spectrum antibiotics and an insulin sliding scale. The priority is to release the pus and debride necrotic tissue. The X-ray changes (osteopenia, osteolysis, sequestra and periostial elevation) suggest there is underlying osteomyelitis (Fig. 47.2). This will also need to be debrided in order to remove all the infection.

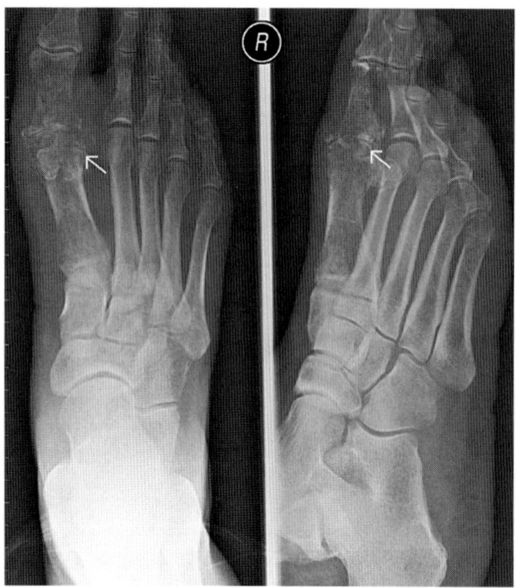

Figure 47.2 Osteomyelitis in the metatarsophalangeal joint of the great toe (arrows).

A duplex scan or intra-arterial angiogram should then be carried out to ascertain whether the blood supply to the foot is compromised and whether any revascularization procedure is necessary.

KEY POINT

- Diabetic feet are at risk of ischemia (progressive distal ischaemia) and neuropathy (sensory, motor and autonomic), and are more prone to infections.

CASE 48: SUDDEN ARM PAIN

History

A 59-year-old woman presents to the emergency department with pain and tingling in the right arm. The pain occurred that morning while she was walking the dog. It was sudden in onset and has improved since arriving in the department. There is no history of trauma and she has had no previous episodes. She is now able to move her fingers, but says they feel numb. Her previous medical history includes intermittent episodes of palpitations for which she is waiting to see a cardiologist.

Examination

The right hand appears pale and feels cool to touch. The radial and ulnar arterial pulses are absent. There is no muscle tenderness in the forearm and she has a full range of active movement in the hand. Sensation is mildly reduced.

INVESTIGATIONS

An urgent angiogram is performed (Fig. 48.1) and an electrocardiogram (ECG, Fig. 48.2).

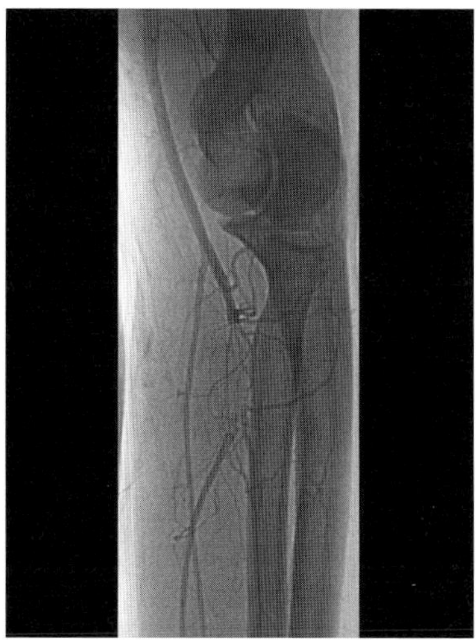

Figure 48.1 Angiogram of the right upper limb.

Questions

- What is the likely diagnosis?
- What is the probable aetiology?
- What other aetiologies do you know for this condition?
- How would you investigate and manage this patient?

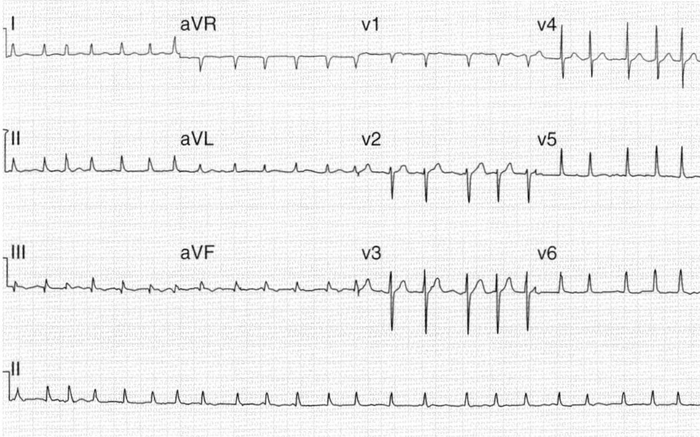

Figure 48.2 Electrocardiogram.

ANSWER 48

This is an acutely ischemic limb secondary to arterial embolism (arrow in Fig. 48.3).

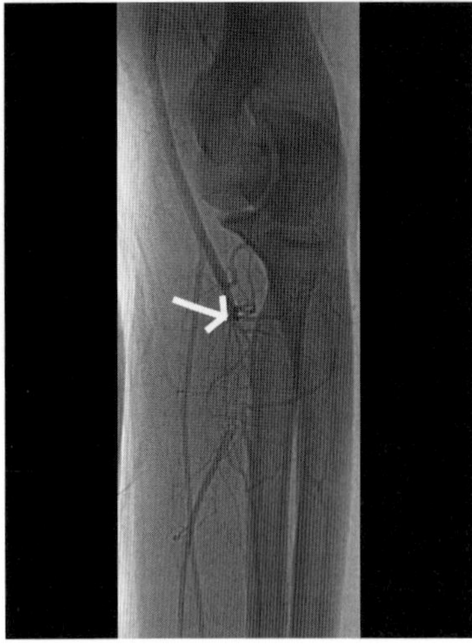

Figure 48.3 Angiogram showing an occlusion of the brachial artery.

The embolus is likely to have originated from the left atrium as the patient has atrial fibrillation (shown on the ECG).

Aetiologies include:

- cardiac arrhythmias: commonly atrial fibrillation
- aneurysmal disease
- procoagulant state caused by underlying malignancy
- thrombophilias
- atrial myxomas.

Investigations aim to determine the aetiology of the embolism and to prepare the patient for theatre:

- full blood count (polycythaemia)
- clotting
- group and save
- ECG (arrhythmias)
- chest X-ray (underlying malignancy).

The patient should be given heparin and resuscitated with intravenous fluids and analgesia. Loss of sensation and paralysis in the affected limb (signs of advanced ischaemia) are indications for urgent embolectomy. A postoperative echocardiogram is arranged if preoperative investigations do not reveal an obvious cause for the embolism. This investigation can detect cardiac thrombus or an atrial myxoma.

KEY POINTS

Signs and symptoms of acute limb ischaemia – six Ps:

- pain
- pulseless
- pallor
- paraesthesia
- perishingly cold
- paralysis.

CASE 49: A NUMB AND PAINFUL HAND

History

A 43-year-old woman presents to the vascular clinic with cramping pain and numbness in the left hand. This morning she has noticed a black patch on the tip of her thumb and index finger. She is a heavy smoker and is on medication for hypertension.

Examination

On examination, the hand is warm and well perfused, with a palpable radial pulse. Allen's test is normal and there is no upper limp neurological deficit. A hard bony swelling is palpable in the supraclavicular fossa. It is not pulsatile and is immobile. A plain radiograph of the thoracic inlet is shown in Fig. 49.1.

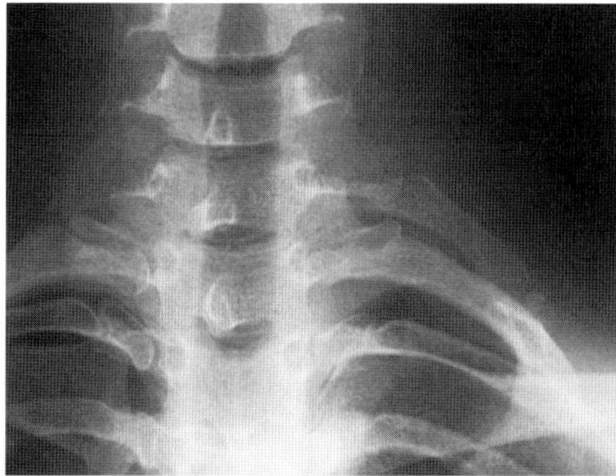

Figure 49.1 Plain anterior-posterior X-ray of the lower cervical spine.

Questions

- What abnormality can be seen in the X-ray?
- What is its incidence in the general population?
- How can the symptoms and signs be explained?
- What is the differential diagnosis?
- What further investigations may be helpful?

ANSWER 49

The X-ray shows a cervical rib (arrow in Fig. 49.2).

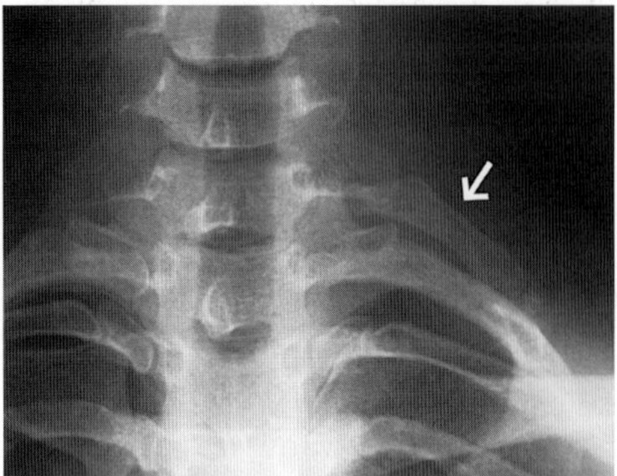

Figure 49.2 Plain X-ray demonstrating a cervical rib (arrow).

Cervical ribs have an incidence of around 0.4 per cent in the general population. The subclavian artery runs over the rib and can be compressed against it. An aneurysm of the artery developing at the point of compression is a rare complication. Thrombus within the aneurysm sac can embolize to the digital arteries and can cause fingertip gangrene or even digital infarction. Thrombosis and occlusion of the subclavian artery can also occur. The brachial plexus runs with the cervical rib, and compression of the T1 nerve root can cause numbness, paraesthesia and weakness. Symptoms maybe relieved by surgical excision of the rib.

The thoracic outlet syndrome can be mimicked by:

- prominent cervical discs
- spinal cord tumours
- cervical spondylosis
- pancoast tumours
- osteoarthritis of the shoulder
- carpal tunnel syndrome
- ulnar neuritis.

An electrocardiogram is required to exclude embolization secondary to cardiac arrhythmias such as atrial fibrillation. A colour Doppler ultrasound scan or an angiogram would determine the presence of a subclavian aneurysm and allow assessment of the distal circulation.

KEY POINTS

- Cervical ribs have an incidence of around 0.4 per cent in the general population.
- Symptoms may be relieved by surgical excision of the cervical rib.

CASE 50: PAIN IN THE CALF ON WALKING

History

A 69-year-old man attends the vascular clinic complaining of a cramping pain in the right calf on walking 150 yards. The pain is worse on an incline and is quickly relieved by rest. The pain is then reproduced after walking the same distance. There is no history of trauma or previous surgery.

Examination

There are no skin changes in the right leg. The right femoral pulse is present but the right popliteal, dorsalis pedis and posterior tibial pulses are absent. A bruit is audible over the right adductor canal. There is no abdominal aortic aneurysm and the rest of the examination is unremarkable.

An angiogram is done and is shown in Fig. 50.1.

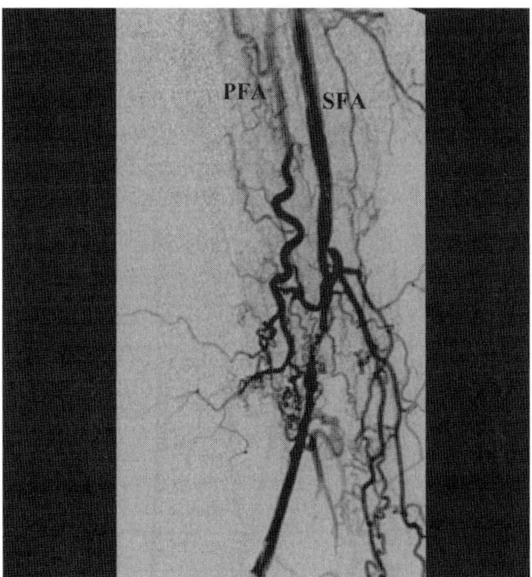

Figure 50.1 Angiogram of the right lower limb. PFA, profunda femoris artery; SFA, superficial femoral artery.

Questions

- What is the most likely diagnosis?
- What are the differential diagnoses for this condition?
- What are the other important points to ascertain from the history?
- What other investigations are required?
- What treatment would you advocate for this man?

ANSWER 50

The most likely diagnosis is intermittent claudication. The angiogram demonstrates a stenosis in the superficial femoral artery at the adductor canal (arrow in Fig. 50.2).

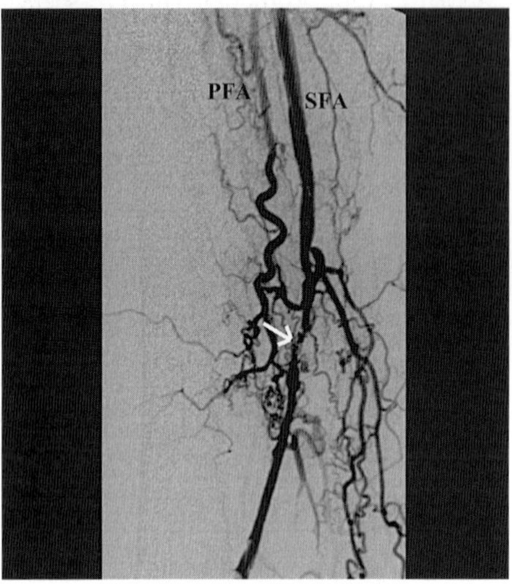

Figure 50.2 Angiogram revealing stenosis in the femoral artery at the adductor canal (arrow).

! Differential diagnoses

- Spinal stenosis
- Nerve root compression
- Venous claudication
- Baker's cyst

The patient should be questioned about risk factors for atherosclerotic disease including cigarette smoking, diabetes, family history, history of cardiac disease, hyperlipidaemia, hyperhomocysteinaemia and hypertension.

Investigations should include ankle–brachial pressure index (ABPI): this is typically <0.9 in patients with claudication; however, calcified vessels (typically in patients with diabetes) may result in an erroneously normal or high ABPI. Other tests include measurement of blood sugar and lipids.

The disease will only progress in 1 in 4 patients with intermittent claudication, therefore, unless the disease is very disabling for the patient, treatment is conservative. This should include reducing the risk of cardiovascular events through secondary prevention:

- smoking cessation
- statins
- antiplatelet drugs
- blood pressure control
- tight diabetes control.

Regular exercise has been shown to increase the claudication distance. In cases that do require intervention, angioplasty and bypass surgery are considered. Angioplasty has a better outcome in single, short stenoses in the common or external iliac arteries.

KEY POINTS

- Risk factors should be addressed as part of the initial management.
- Patients should be encouraged to exercise to improve the collateral circulation.

CASE 51: LOWER LIMB ULCERATION

History

A 50-year-old man presents to the vascular clinic with an ulcer on the lower aspect of the left leg. It appeared 3 months ago following minor trauma to the leg and has grown in size steadily. There is no other past medical history of note.

Examination

There is an ulcer, shown in Fig. 51.1, with slough and exudate at the base. There is surrounding dark pigmentation. Examination of the rest of the leg shows varicose veins in the long saphenous distribution.

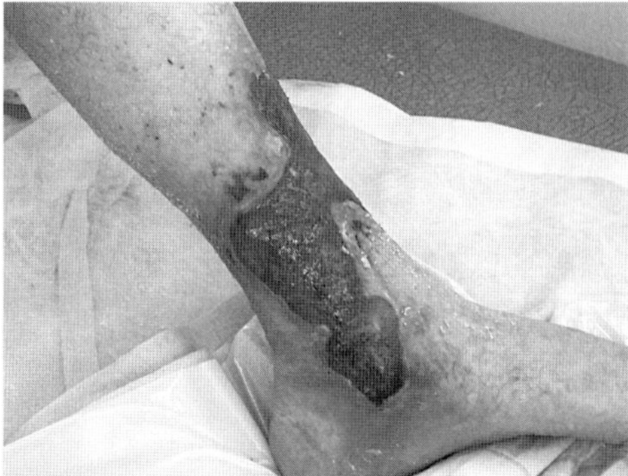

Figure 51.1 Venous ulceration.

Questions

- What is the definition of an ulcer?
- What are the causes of ulceration?
- What else should be included in the examination and investigation for lower limb ulceration?
- What does the management of a venous ulcer involve?
- How should the patient be managed once the ulcer has healed?

ANSWER 51

An ulcer is the dissolution of an epithelial surface. This patient has venous ulceration. The ulcer is situated in the medial gaiter region. The edges slope and the base has healthy tissue. The surrounding skin changes support a venous aetiology.

! Causes of leg ulceration

- Venous
- Arterial
- Mixed venous/arterial
- Diabetic: underlying aetiology neuropathic/arterial or mixture of both
- Rheumatoid
- Scleroderma
- Sickle cell
- Syphilitic
- Pyoderma gangrenosum

During examination, peripheral pulses should be palpated and Doppler pressures obtained. Investigations include full blood count and erythrocyte sedimentation rate, autoantibodies (if there is a possibility of rheumatoid vasculitis) and blood glucose levels.

The mainstay of treatment for venous ulcers is calf pump compression using multi-layered bandages applied to the lower leg. The ulcer is inspected weekly to ensure that it is healing, and bandages are re-applied. An ulcer that fails to heal with these measures may benefit from surgical debridement and the application of a mesh skin graft. Malignant transformation (Marjolin's ulcer) can develop in a long-standing, non-healing venous ulcer.

Once the ulcer has healed the superficial and deep veins of the leg should be assessed using a duplex Doppler scan. Saphenous vein surgery should be considered if there is evidence of sapheno-femoral or sapheno-popliteal reflux with patent deep veins. This can prevent recurrences. Patients who do not undergo surgery should wear graduated elastic support stockings to prevent recurrence.

KEY POINTS

- Venous ulceration should be treated with compression bandaging.
- Caution should be taken in patients with peripheral arterial disease.

CASE 52: PUNCHED OUT ULCERATION

History

A 69-year-old retired plumber presents to the emergency department complaining of a painful, non-healing wound on the right lower leg. He knocked his leg on a supermarket trolley 4 weeks ago and the wound has grown in size since then. Over the past 6 months he has been getting pain in both his calves after walking approximately 10 yards. He is on medication for hypercholesterolaemia and hypertension. He had a myocardial infarction 5 years ago. He smokes 25 cigarettes each day.

Examination

There is a 4 × 5 cm punched-out ulcer on the lateral aspect of the right lower leg with some surrounding erythema. In addition there is a small ulcer between the third and fourth toe. The right foot feels cooler than the left, but capillary return is not diminished. There is a full range of movement in the right foot and sensation is intact. The femoral pulse is palpable on both sides, but no popliteal, dorsalis pedis or posterior tibial pulses are present on either side.

INVESTIGATIONS

An angiogram is done and is shown in Fig. 52.1.

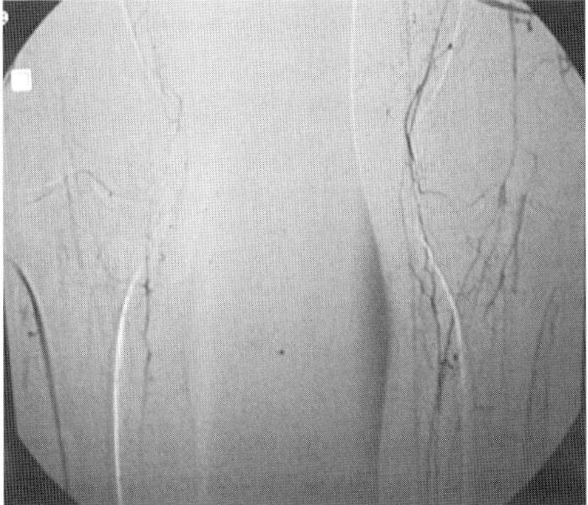

Figure 52.1

Questions

- What is the likely aetiology of the ulceration?
- What does the angiogram reveal?
- What other investigations need to be carried out?
- What are the treatment options?

ANSWER 52

The limb is ischaemic with tissue loss secondary to arterial insufficiency. The most common cause of ischaemia is atherosclerosis. This patient's angiogram reveals that all the major vessels in both legs are occluded from the level of the popliteal artery downwards. Multiple small collaterals are seen on both sides.

The investigations should include:

- ankle–brachial pressure index: this is related to the severity of symptoms but may be inaccurate in diabetic patients:
  - 1.0: normal
  - 0.5–0.9: claudication
  - <0.4: rest pain
  - <0.2: risk of limb loss
- blood tests including full blood count, urea and electrolytes, glucose
- electrocardiogram
- angiography: intra-arterial angiography can be used to delineate stenoses and treat those amenable to angioplasty. Computerized tomography and magnetic resonance angiography are alternative imaging modalities.

It is important to distinguish arterial from venous ulceration, as use of compression to treat the former type of ulcer is contraindicated. Patients with tissue loss require intervention. Short, single stenoses in the vessels above the inguinal ligament are amenable to angioplasty. Below the inguinal ligament the results are not as good and the patient may be best served by bypass surgery. Similarly, multiple stenoses, long stenoses (>10 cm) and calcified vessels are best treated with a bypass. Investigations may show that the stenoses are not suitable for either angioplasty or bypass surgery (i.e. absence of a suitable distal vessel to bypass onto), in which case a primary amputation may be the end result.

KEY POINTS

Medical treatments should not be neglected. These include:

- pain control: opiate analgesia is often required
- antiplatelet agents: e.g. aspirin, clopidogrel
- lipid-lowering agents: e.g. statins
- anticoagulants: e.g. low-molecular-weight/unfractionated heparin.

CASE 53: REST PAIN IN THE LOWER LIMB

History

A 70-year-old man presents to the emergency department complaining of a dull pain in the dorsum of the right foot for the past 6 weeks. The pain is worse at night, waking him from sleep, and is relieved by hanging his leg over the edge of the bed. For the past week he has been sleeping in a chair to alleviate the pain. He is known to have hypertension and hypercholesterolaemia. His past history includes coronary artery bypass grafting 6 years ago. He lives with his wife and is fully independent.

Examination

The right foot has a red tinge and is swollen. The right little toe is dusky. The right foot feels cool when compared with the left, with delayed capillary refill. The femoral pulse is palpable on both sides. Pulses are palpable on the left leg, but pulses below the femoral are absent on the right. The ankle–brachial pressure index measures 0.9 on the left and 0.35 on the right.

The patient is admitted for urgent angiography (Fig. 53.1).

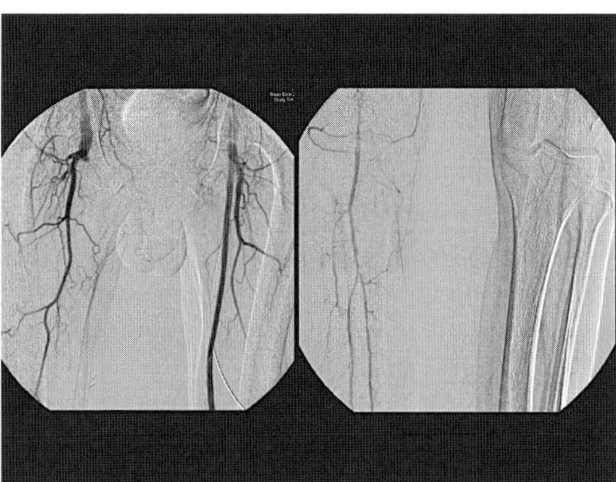

Figure 53.1 Angiogram of the right lower limb.

Questions

- How do you explain the symptoms and signs?
- A decision is made to carry out arterial reconstruction – what choices of graft materials are available?
- What are the complications of surgery?

ANSWER 53

Pain in the foot that is worse at night and is relieved by dependence is classical of ischaemic rest pain and is the result of poor tissue perfusion and oxygenation. An ankle–brachial pressure index of 0.35 is compatible. Discolouration of the toe suggests impending gangrene. The angiogram reveals occlusion of the superficial femoral artery on the right (Fig. 53.2). The popliteal artery reforms at the level of the knee via collateral vessels. This patient should be considered for a femoral-popliteal bypass graft.

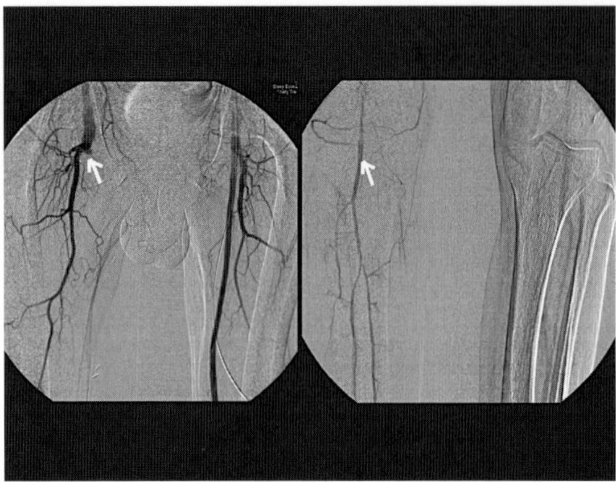

Figure 53.2 Arterial angiogram showing occlusion of the right superficial femoral artery and the popliteal artery reforming at the knee (arrows).

The patient should firstly be admitted and made comfortable using opiate analgesia. He should be treated with low-molecular-weight or unfractionated heparin, pending investigation and treatment.

The material of choice for bypass grafting is autogenous vein. The long saphenous vein is most widely used but arm veins/the short saphenous vein are other options if the long saphenous vein has already been used (e.g. previous bypass, coronary artery grafting) or is small in calibre. Other options include umbilical vein allografts or prosthetic grafts (e.g. Dacron, polytetrafluoroethylene). The long-term patency of prosthetic grafts is inferior compared with autogenous vein.

! Complications of bypass surgery

- *Early*:
  - haemorrhage
  - graft thrombosis
  - compartment syndrome
  - deep vein thrombosis/pulmonary embolism
  - cardiorespiratory complications
- *Late*:
  - graft stenosis/occlusion
  - delayed wound healing
  - graft sepsis
  - anastomotic false aneurysms
  - limb loss

KEY POINTS

- Rest pain indicates inadequate tissue perfusion.
- Urgent investigation and treatment is required to salvage the limb.

CASE 54: POSTOPERATIVE LIMB SWELLING

History

You are asked to review a 68-year-old woman on the ward. She had an anterior resection for a rectal tumour 5 days ago. Postoperative recovery has been unremarkable and she has started to eat and drink and opened her bowels today. You have been asked to examine her as she is complaining of pain and swelling of the left leg. There is no history of trauma to the leg.

Examination

Her temperature is 37.5°C and her pulse rate is 99/min. The abdomen is soft and non-tender. The left leg is swollen to mid-thigh, with erythema of the skin. The calf feels warm and is tender to touch. The foot pulses are normal.

INVESTIGATIONS

		Normal
Haemoglobin	11.5 g/dL	11.5–16.0 g/dL
White cell count	16.7 $\times 10^9$/L	4.0–11.0 $\times 10^9$/L
Platelets	360 $\times 10^9$/L	150–400 $\times 10^9$/L
Sodium	143 mmol/L	135–145 mmol/L
Potassium	4.6 mmol/L	3.5–5.0 mmol/L
Urea	9.5 mmol/L	2.5–6.7 mmmol/L
Creatinine	71 μmol/L	(44–80 μmol/L
C-reactive protein	100 mg/L	<5 mg/L

Questions

- What is the most likely diagnosis? What are the differentials?
- What investigation should be carried out next?
- What are the risk factors associated with this condition?
- How should this condition be treated?
- What are the long-term sequelae of this condition?

ANSWER 54

The most likely diagnosis is a deep vein thombosis (DVT). Clinical examination is notoriously inaccurate for making the diagnosis, as the degree of swelling and pain varies and patients can be symptomless.

! Differential diagnoses

- Cellulitis
- Lymphangitis
- Soft tissue injury
- Lymphoedema
- Haematoma
- Arterial insufficiency
- Ruptured Baker's cyst

A normal D-dimer assay (fibrin degradation products) would usually be used to exclude a diagnosis of DVT, but is not useful in this case as the recent surgery means that it will be positive regardless. The diagnosis is best confirmed using duplex ultrasonography of the deep veins.

! Risk factors for deep vein thrombosis

- Age
- Bed rest
- Pregnancy
- Oral contraceptive pill
- Major surgery
- Medical
- Major trauma
- Burns
- Lower-extremity fractures
- Haematological
- Thrombocytosis
- Polycythaemia
- Protein S deficiency
- Protein C deficiency
- Antithrombin III deficiency
- Factor V Leiden

Anticoagulation is the mainstay of treatment, aimed at preventing extension of the thrombus and reducing the risk of pulmonary embolism. Therapeutic low-molecular-weight heparin and warfarin are commenced at the same time. Heparin is stopped when the international normalized ratio becomes therapeutic. Some authorities do not treat DVT confined to the calf because of the very low risk of pulmonary embolism.

DVT can result in venous hypertension, and long-term consequences include the post-thrombotic syndrome which consists of leg pain, swelling, lipodermatosclerosis and ulceration.

 **KEY POINTS**

- Treatment should be commenced once a DVT has been diagnosed clinically.
- The diagnosis is confirmed with ultrasound.

CASE 55: INVESTIGATION OF A SWOLLEN LIMB

History

A 43-year-old Caucasian woman presents to the surgical outpatients with right leg swelling. This first appeared 3 weeks ago and has gradually increased such that she finds it difficult to put on her shoe. She is otherwise symptomless. There is no history of trauma to the limb. Apart from a tonsillectomy as a child, there is no past history of note. She is on the oral contraceptive pill.

Examination

There is unilateral swelling of the right lower leg from the foot to just above the knee (Fig. 55.1). There is no associated erythema and no stigmata of venous disease. The oedema pits when the skin is pressed. All pulses in the leg are palpable. The general examination is otherwise unremarkable.

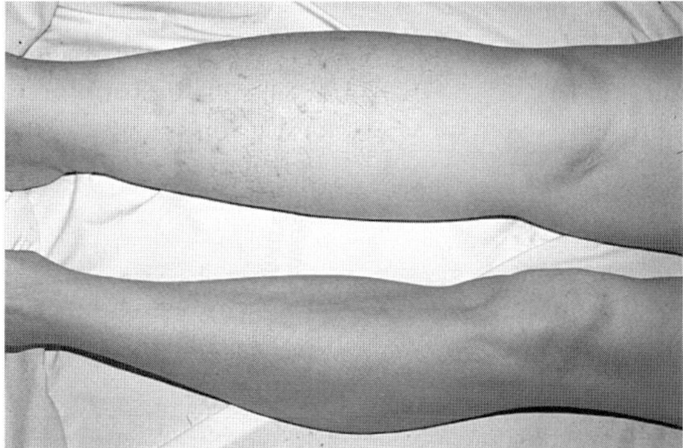

Figure 55.1 Unilateral right leg swelling.

Questions

- What is the differential diagnosis of leg swelling?
- What investigations are required?
- What are the two most likely diagnoses in this patient?
- What are the treatment options?

ANSWER 55

The common causes of unilateral limb swelling are:

- long-standing venous disease (e.g. post-thrombotic syndrome)
- acute deep vein thrombosis
- lymphoedema
- extrinsic pressure (e.g. pregnancy, tumour, retroperitoneal fibrosis)
- Klippel–Trénaunay syndrome
- lipoedema
- disuse/hysterical oedema.

Bilateral symmetrical limb swelling is usually caused by systemic factors such as:

- heart failure
- renal failure
- liver cirrhosis
- hypoproteinaemia
- hereditary angioedema.

Useful investigations include:

- blood tests: full blood count, urea and electrolytes, liver function test, albumin
- electrocardiogram/echocardiography
- abdominal ultrasound
- duplex scanning of deep and superficial veins if a venous cause is suspected
- isotope lymphography
- contrast lymphography, if diagnosis of lymphoedema equivocal.

The most likely diagnoses are either deep vein thrombosis or lymphoedema. Lymphoedema is either primary or secondary. Secondary causes include:

- surgical excision of local lymph nodes
- radiotherapy to local lymph nodes
- tumour infiltrating the lymphatics
- trauma
- filiriasis
- lymphoedema artifacta: patient tying a tourniquet around the limb.

In lymphoedema, the vast majority of patients (>90 per cent) are treated conservatively. Interstitial fluid is driven from the limb using intermittent pneumatic compression devices. Compression is maintained using elastic stockings. Massage of the leg may also be beneficial. Patients are advised to elevate the leg when possible and to be vigilant for signs of cellulitis which should be treated promptly. Diuretics are not useful.

Debulking operations (e.g. Charles and Homan's reduction) are only considered for a selected few patients where the function of the limb is impaired or those with recurrent attacks of severe cellulitis.

KEY POINT

- The majority of patients with lymphoedema are managed conservatively.

CASE 56: VARICOSE VEINS

History

You are asked to see a 47-year-old hairdresser in the vascular clinic. She has been complaining of pain in the right leg on prolonged standing and has noticed unsightly, distended veins in that leg for the past 2 years. For the past 3 months she has also had itching of the skin just below the knee with a red patch in that area. She is currently on treatment for hypertension with no other past history of note. She has two children.

Examination

A distended vein can be felt in the medial aspect of the mid-thigh running down to the knee. There are numerous varicosities around and below the knee. There is an erythematous patch of skin approximately 3 cm in diameter overlying one of the below-knee varicosities. A thrill is palpable at the sapheno-femoral junction when the patient coughs. Foot pulses are strongly palpable.

Questions

- What is the most likely diagnosis?
- What information would the Trendelenburg test provide?
- What is the significance of the erythematous patch of skin?
- What imaging studies would you consider?
- What are the possible complications if left untreated?

ANSWER 56

This patient has varicose veins in the distribution of the long saphenous vein, a common condition that is more common in women. Working as a hairdresser involves prolonged standing, which increases venous hydrostatic pressure leading to distension of the veins and secondary valve incompetence within the superficial venous system.

The Trendelenburg test can confirm superficial as opposed to deep-vein incompetence and identify the point of incompetence along the superficial system. The leg is elevated to collapse all the veins and pressure is applied on the long saphenous vein just below the sapheno-femoral junction. The patient then stands up, and if the distal varicosities remain empty the point of reflux from the deep to the superficial system has been identified. If the varicosities fill, then the procedure is repeated, this time applying the pressure at a lower point until the point of reflux is identified.

The itching erythematous patch represents varicose eczema and is an indication for operative intervention.

Imaging identifies all areas of reflux and obstruction within the superficial and deep-venous system. Duplex ultrasound is now the standard imaging modality for this purpose. Alternatives include contrast varicography/venography and magnetic resonance imaging.

Sequelae of varicose veins

- Pain
- Leg swelling
- Bleeding
- Eczema
- Skin ulceration

KEY POINTS

- Further skin changes may be prevented with surgical correction of the superficial venous reflux disease.
- Surgery on the superficial venous system should be avoided in patients with an incompetent deep venous system.

UROLOGY

CASE 57: TESTICULAR PAIN

History

A 16-year-old boy attends the emergency department complaining of sudden onset of right testicular pain. The pain woke him from his sleep and has persisted over the last 3 h. His mother says that he has vomited once. His previous medical history includes a similar event a year ago, but on that occasion the pain subsided quickly. He is asthmatic and uses a salbutamol inhaler.

Examination

On examination the left hemi-scrotum feels normal but the right side is acutely swollen and tender on palpation. The testicle is elevated when compared to the other side and has an abnormal horizontal lie. The abdomen is soft and non-tender. His blood pressure is 130/84 mmHg and the pulse rate is 110/min. The cremasteric reflex is absent.

INVESTIGATIONS

Urinalysis is clear.

Questions

- What is the diagnosis?
- What should you consider in the differential?
- What is the management in this case?

ANSWER 57

This boy has testicular torsion until proven otherwise. It is likely that a year ago he had an episode of intermittent torsion with spontaneous detorsion. Testicular torsion is actually torsion of the spermatic cord and not of the testis. This results in irreversible ischaemia to the testicular parenchyma which can occur within 4–6 h of cord torsion. The presentation can vary and includes vague loin or groin pain as well as scrotal signs and symptoms. There may be a history of excessive physical activity or trauma. It is more common between late childhood (post-puberty) and early adulthood.

Normally, the tunica vaginalis envelops the body of the testis and only part of the epididymis (which is usually fixed), and the testis is unable to twist. In cases of torsion, there is an abnormal amount of free space between the parietal and visceral layers of the tunica vaginalis which encompasses the testis, epididymis and the cord for a variable distance. This free space allows the now hypermobile testis and epididymis to rise in the scrotum and twist. This accounts for the abnormal horizontal lie of the testis ('bell clapper deformity'). If the presentation is delayed, an acute hydrocoele may develop making examination difficult, and the scrotum may appear erythematous. Surgical exploration is essential if torsion is considered. Urinalysis is often negative and the diagnosis should be made clinically.

! Differential diagnoses

- torsion of the appendix testis
- torsion of the appendix epididymis
- epididymo-orchitis
- infected hydrocoele
- testicular rupture
- strangulated inguinal hernia
- a bleed into a tumour

In torsion of the appendix testis, the tenderness is usually localized above the upper pole of the testis and may be accompanied by the 'blue dot' sign, which represents necrosis in the appendix. Hydrocoeles may be tender if large and will transilluminate. If a patient is suspected of having epididymo-orchitis, the urine should be screened for infection. There may also be a history of urethral discharge or urinary symptoms such as frequency or dysuria.

KEY POINTS

- If testicular torsion is suspected, surgical exploration should be carried out as soon as possible.
- Irreversible ischaemia of the testis occurs after approximately 6 h.

CASE 58: LEFT LOIN PAIN

History

A 33-year-old female office worker presents to the emergency department complaining of severe left-sided abdominal pain. The pain woke her in the early hours of the morning and has persisted throughout the day. She is unable to keep still and has vomited bilious material on five occasions. She reports no diarrhoea or rectal bleeding. Previous medical history includes appendicectomy and irritable bowel syndrome. She has had a recent colonoscopy which was normal. She takes mebeverine for irritable bowel syndrome and multivitamin tablets. She smokes 15 cigarettes per day.

Examination

On examination she has a temperature of 37°C, a blood pressure of 125/88 mmHg and pulse rate of 96/min. There is marked left loin tenderness, but the rest of the abdomen is non-tender. Heart sounds are normal and the chest is clear.

INVESTIGATIONS

		Normal
Haemoglobin	12.6 g/dL	11.5–16.0 g/dL
White cell count	12.8 × 10^9/L	4.0–11.0 × 10^9/L
Platelets	254 × 10^9/L	150–400 × 10^9/L
Sodium	141 mmol/L	135–145 mmol/L
Potassium	4.2 mmol/L	3.5–5.0 mmol/L
Urea	5.0 mmol/L	2.5–6.7 mmmol/L
Creatinine	62 μmol/L	44–80 μmol/L

Urinalysis:
Protein: negative
Nitrites: negative
Leucocytes: +1
Blood: +4
Glucose: negative
Human chorionic gonadotrophin: negative

Questions

- What is the likely diagnosis?
- What investigation would you like to do to confirm your diagnosis?
- What are the indications for admitting this patient?
- What is the initial management?

ANSWER 58

The combination of left loin pain and microscopic haematuria, in the absence of abdominal peritonism, suggests a diagnosis of renal/ureteric colic. In 10–15 per cent of cases of renal colic, the dipstick will be negative for blood. The differential diagnosis includes pyelonephritis, diverticulitis, bowel obstruction, peptic ulcer disease and gynaecological conditions such as ectopic pregnancy, torted ovarian cyst or tubo-ovarian abscess. In addition to the above, on the right side, appendicitis and biliary colic should also be considered. In an older patient it is important to exclude a ruptured abdominal aortic aneurysm.

The pain of renal colic is caused by the distension of the ureter or collecting system from an obstructing calculus. The pain may radiate from loin to groin and to the tip of the penis in males and to the labia in females. Calculi may also irritate the bladder, causing urgency, frequency and strangury.

Approximately 90 per cent of urinary tract calculi are radio-opaque and may be seen on a plain kidney, ureter, bladder (KUB) X-ray. The presence of a calculus is often obscured by overlying bowel gas. An intravenous urethrogram (IVU) is used to confirm the diagnosis and the level of the obstruction. Intravenous contrast is administered with repeat KUB X-rays at 5 and 20 min, with a post-micturition film, usually at one hour. A further delayed KUB may be required to detect the level of obstruction if it is not seen on the original X-ray series. An increasingly popular alternative to IVU is a computerized tomography (CT) KUB (performed without contrast), which is more sensitive in detecting all types of urinary tract calculi (with the exception of indinavir stones), with the added benefit of screening for other pathology.

Indications for admitting the patient include:

- complete obstruction: unilateral/bilateral
- pain not controlled with simple analgesia
- evidence of sepsis, e.g. pyrexia, raised white cell count or signs and symptoms of septic shock

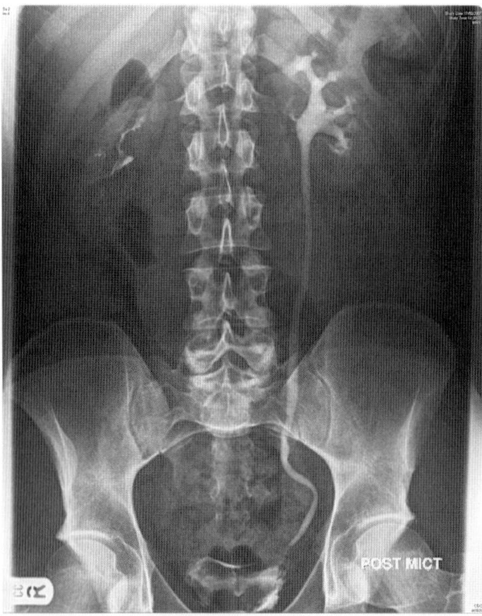

Figure 58.1 Left sided distal vesico-ureteric calculus causing a standing column of contrast (1 h film and post-micturition).

- calculi in a solitary kidney
- deranged renal function.

The analgesic of choice is rectal diclofenac, although in some cases opiates will be required. Fluids should be given and in cases of suspected infection antibiotics with good gram-negative cover administered.

The IVU in Fig. 58.1 is a delayed post-micturition film revealing a standing column of contrast down to the level of the left vesico-ureteric junction, indicating that this is the level of obstruction.

KEY POINTS

- Haematuria is present in 90 per cent of cases of renal colic.
- Approximately 90 per cent of calculi are visible on a plain X-ray.

CASE 59: LOWER URINARY TRACT SYMPTOMS

History

A 71-year-old man has been referred to the urology outpatient clinic with a history of urinary frequency, nocturia and some post-micturition dribbling. He has occasional urgency. He suffers with osteoarthritis of his left hip and uses a walking stick. He has angina, hypertension and hypercholesteraemia. He is an ex-smoker and lives with his wife. His younger brother had prostate cancer and underwent a radical prostatectomy at the age of 65 years. He is anxious to get his prostate-specific antigen (PSA) tested as he is concerned about prostate cancer.

Examination

Abdominal examination is unremarkable. The bladder is not palpable and the genitalia are normal with no evidence of stenosis of the urethral meatus or phimosis. Digital rectal examination confirms a moderately enlarged smooth prostate gland.

INVESTIGATIONS

		Normal
Haemoglobin	14.2 g/dL	11.5–16.0 g/dL
White cell count	6.6×10^9/L	$4.0–11.0 \times 10^9$/L
Platelets	376×10^9/L	$150–400 \times 10^9$/L
Sodium	138 mmol/L	135–145 mmol/L
Potassium	4.1 mmol/L	3.5–5.0 mmol/L
Urea	4.2 mmol/L	2.5–6.7 mmmol/L
Creatinine	79 μmol/L	44–80 μmol/L
PSA: 6.1 ng/mL		
International Prostate Symptom Score (IPSS) score: 21		
Urinalysis: NAD (nothing abnormal detected)		
Flow rate:		
Voided volume	212 mL	
$\dot{Q}_{max}$ (maximal flow rate)	12 mL/s	
Post-void residual volume	91 mL	

Questions

- What are the causes of an elevated PSA?
- How would you classify this patient's symptoms?
- What is the likely diagnosis in this patient?
- What treatment would you recommend?

ANSWER 59

Prostate-specific antigen is a glycoprotein enzyme produced by the prostate gland. Its function is to liquefy the ejaculate and to aid sperm motility. In symptomless men appropriate counselling is required prior to performing a PSA blood test. A raised PSA may be caused by benign prostatic hyperplasia (BPH), prostatitis, urinary tract infection, urinary retention, instrumentation (e.g. catheterization), biopsy, a transurethral resection of the prostate (TURP) or by prostate cancer. Prostate cancer screening is not currently of proven benefit, although several trials are investigating its value at present. PSA values vary with age, reflecting the effect of BPH on the prostate gland. Normal ranges are outlined in Table 59.1.

Table 59.1 PSA values

Age (years)	PSA ng/mL
All	<4
40–49	<2.5
50–59	<3.5
60–69	<4.5
>70	<6.5

This patient has lower urinary tract symptoms (LUTS) which are classically divided into two groups:

- *obstructive*: weakness of urinary stream, hesitancy, terminal dribbling, intermittency, feeling of incomplete bladder emptying
- *irritative*: urinary urgency, frequency, nocturia and incontinence.

Patients with bladder outflow obstruction may present with obstructive symptoms alone or in conjunction with irritative symptoms. The irritative symptoms are secondary to the obstruction which leads to changes in the bladder causing bladder overactivity. In this case the patient has LUTS secondary to BPH. Organizing a PSA for LUTS alone is reasonable, but in this case the patient has other risk factors – family history and his age. Other indications to organize a PSA blood test include an abnormal digital rectal examination, progressive back pain, unexplained weight loss and prostate cancer monitoring.

Baseline LUTS can be measured using the International Prostate Symptom Score (IPSS; range 0–35), a symptom index questionnaire. This is useful in monitoring the response to treatment. In this case he has moderate symptoms. Other factors that point to the diagnosis of BPH include his low maximal flow rate (normal in males >30 mL/s; females >40 mL/s) and his elevated post-micturition residual volume, which indicates incomplete bladder emptying (another feature of significant bladder outflow obstruction).

Treatment options include watchful waiting (periodic monitoring, lifestyle advice), medical therapy (alpha-blockers and/or 5-alpha reductase inhibitors) and surgery (TURP).

KEY POINTS

- The serum PSA may be raised in benign disease.
- Patients should be counselled prior to PSA testing.

CASE 60: RIGHT FLANK PAIN WITH URINARY SYMPTOMS

History

A 28-year-old female presents to the emergency department complaining of right-sided abdominal pain for the previous 10 days. She initially saw her general practitioner with this problem about a week before and was prescribed antibiotics. Her symptoms initially improved but have now worsened. She has had rigors at home today and her anxious partner organized for her to come into hospital. She has vomited once. Her previous medical history includes an appendicectomy and an episode of pelvic inflammatory disease. She is a smoker. There is no history of diarrhoea, but the patient describes some soreness on micturition and has a clear vaginal discharge.

Examination

Her temperature is 38.7°C, blood pressure 129/76 mmHg and her pulse rate is 115/min. There is tenderness on the right side of the abdomen and right flank. The rest of the abdomen is unremarkable. The heart sounds are normal and on auscultation of the chest there appears to be some dullness to percussion and reduced air entry in the right lower zone.

INVESTIGATIONS

		Normal
Haemoglobin	13.4 g/dL	11.5–16.0 g/dL
White cell count	18.8 × 10^9/L	4.0–11.0 × 10^9/L
Platelets	254 × 10^9/L	150–400 × 10^9/L
Sodium	140 mmol/L	135–145 mmol/L
Potassium	4.4 mmol/L	3.5–5.0 mmol/L
Urea	5.1 mmol/L	2.5–6.7 mmmol/L
Creatinine	78 μmol/L	44–80 μmol/L
Urinalysis:		
Protein: +1		
Leucocytes: +2		
Nitrites: +ve		
Blood: +1		

Questions

- What is the most likely diagnosis and what other conditions must be considered in the differential?
- What investigations are necessary?
- What is the initial management?

ANSWER 60

This patient appears to have a right-sided acute pyelonephritis, based on her elevated white blood cell count, temperature, urinalysis and right-sided flank pain. However, it is important to consider a gynaecological cause given her previous history, but in this case the positive dipstick points to pathology in the urinary tract. Other conditions that need to be considered include appendicitis (but in this case she has already had her appendix removed), acute cholecystitis, right basal pneumonia and pancreatitis. In an elderly patient, diverticulitis should be considered for pain on the left side.

Acute pyelonephritis is an acute inflammatory reaction involving the renal parenchyma and collecting system. *Escherichia coli* is the commonest infecting organism and accounts for approximately 80 per cent of cases. The infection usually ascends from the distal urinary tract and bladder and less commonly comes through the bloodstream. It may be bilateral.

! Predisposing causes

- Urinary tract obstruction
- Renal calculi
- Diabetes mellitus
- Pregnancy
- Anatomical/congenital anomalies e.g. pelvi-ureteric junction obstruction
- Vesicoureteric reflux
- Neurogenic bladder
- Immunosuppression
- Long-term urinary catheter

Initial investigations include a urine dipstick, mid-stream urine, blood cultures, full blood count and urea and electrolytes. A plain radiograph of the kidneys, ureters and bladder is helpful to assess for urinary tract calculi. A renal ultrasound scan provides information on renal calculi and whether a hydronephrosis is present as a result of an obstructed urinary system. The patient should be started on intravenous antibiotics with good gram-negative and common gram-positive cover. In less severe cases, management can be on an outpatient basis with a prolonged course of oral antibiotics.

KEY POINTS

- *E. coli* is the commonest infective organism.
- Recurrent infection requires further investigation.

CASE 61: RENAL MASS

History

A 61-year-old male presented to his general practitioner (GP) complaining of intermittent left-sided loin pain for 2 months. An ultrasound scan of the urinary tract was organized, which showed a large central mass in the left kidney. His previous medical history included a recent diagnosis of hypertension, hypothyroidism and non-insulin-dependent diabetes mellitus. He currently takes thyroxine 100 μg od, bendrofluazide 2.5 mg od and metformin 850 mg bd. He lives alone and drinks 5–10 units of alcohol per week. He is a lifelong smoker.

Examination

His temperature is 37°C, his blood pressure is 165/99 mmHg and his pulse is 84/min. Heart sounds are normal and his chest is clear. He has a soft non-tender abdomen with no palpable masses. A left sided varicocoele is present. Digital rectal examination is unremarkable.

INVESTIGATIONS

Urinalysis:
Blood: ++
Leucocytes: negative
Protein: negative
Glucose: +

Ultrasound of the urinary tract: there is a solid central mass measuring 3.6 cm in the left kidney. The right kidney appears normal. There is no evidence of pelvi-calyceal dilatation or calculi on either side. The bladder was not filled and was therefore difficult to examine.

Questions

- What investigation is now required?
- Can you explain why the patient may have a varicocoele?
- Do you know of a genetic condition that may predispose individuals to renal cell carcinoma?
- Why may the patient be hypertensive?

ANSWER 61

The patient has been found to have a renal mass on ultrasound scan. The most likely diagnosis is renal cell carcinoma and the patient now requires a contrast computerized tomography (CT) scan of the abdomen and pelvis to confirm the diagnosis and to stage his disease. A chest X-ray should also be organized to screen for chest metastases (if a CT of the chest is not performed at the same time of his staging). Approximately one-quarter to one-third of patients with renal cell carcinomas have metastases at presentation.

The venous drainage from the testes (pampiniform plexus) is into the gonadal (testicular) veins. On the left, the gonadal vein drains into the left renal vein and on the right the vein drains directly into the inferior vena cava. Tumours extending into the left renal vein will obstruct the venous drainage from the left testicle, leading to a left-sided varicocoele.

The commonest genetic abnormality associated with renal cell carcinoma is von Hippel–Lindau syndrome. This is an autosomal dominant disease characterized by phaeochromocytoma, pancreatic and renal cysts, cerebellar haemangioblastoma and the development of renal cell carcinoma which is often bilateral. Lifelong follow-up is required and nephron-sparing surgery employed in view of the recurrent nature of the disease.

Other non-genetic aetiological factors associated with renal cell carcinoma include:

- smoking
- anatomical: horseshoe kidney; polycystic disease; cystic disease of dialysis
- hypertension
- obesity
- environmental: cadmium, asbestos exposure, phenacitin (analgesic)
- low social class.

The classic presenting triad of loin pain, a mass and haematuria only occurs in about 10 per cent of patients. More commonly one of these features appears in isolation. Other presentations include left-sided varicocoele (5 per cent) and paraneoplastic syndromes (10–40 per cent).

! Paraneoplastic syndromes

- *Endocrine* (ectopic hormone production):
  - erythropoietin: polycythaemia
  - renin: hypertension
  - insulin: hypoglycaemia
  - adrenocorticotrophic hormone (ACTH): Cushing's syndrome
  - parathyroid hormone: hypercalcaemia
  - gonadotrophins: gynaecomastia, amenorrhea, reduced libido, baldness
- *Haematological*: anaemia
- *Metabolic*: pyrexia

KEY POINTS

- The classic presenting triad of loin pain, a mass and haematuria only occurs in a small proportion of patients.
- Patients may present with a paraneoplastic syndrome.

CASE 62: HAEMATURIA

History

A 60-year-old woman attends the emergency department complaining of a 3-week history of blood in the urine. She has also noted the passage of some small blood clots. She has had an intermittent urinary stream for the last 24 h and complains of pain in the suprapubic region on voiding. She has been complaining of urinary frequency and urgency for the last 6 months. She smokes 10 cigarettes per day and takes warfarin for atrial fibrillation.

Examination

On examination of the abdomen there is some minor suprapubic tenderness, and a palpable bladder. The rest of the examination is unremarkable. Her pulse rate is 100/min and the blood pressure is 105/70 mmHg.

INVESTIGATIONS

		Normal
Haemoglobin	8.2 g/dL	11.5–16.0 g/dL
White cell count	13.6 × 10^9/L	4.0–11.0 × 10^9/L
Platelets	400 × 10^9/L	150–400 × 10^9/L
Sodium	134 mmol/L	135–145 mmol/L
Potassium	4.8 mmol/L	3.5–5.0 mmol/L
Urea	6.7 mmol/L	2.5–6.7 mmmol/L
Creatinine	92 μmol/L	44–80 μmol/L
International normalized ratio (INR)	2.2 IU	1 IU

Questions

- What is the differential diagnosis and what is the most important diagnosis to exclude in this woman?
- What factors are relevant in taking a history in this case?
- What is the initial management in this woman?

ANSWER 62

Haematuria can be classified as either macroscopic (frank) or microscopic (picked up on dipstick testing).

! Causes of haematuria

- *Kidneys*: neoplasia (benign, e.g. angiomyolipoma; malignant, e.g. renal cell carcinoma), polycystic kidneys, calculi, pyelonephritis, tuberculosis, glomerulonephritis or immunoglobulin A (IgA) nephropathy
- *Ureter*: transitional cell carcinoma or calculi
- *Bladder*: neoplasia, e.g. transitional cell carcinoma, squamous cell carcinoma, calculi, inflammatory or infective causes – cystitis, schistosomiasis
- *Prostate*: prostatitis, carcinoma or benign prostatic hyperplasia
- *Urethra*: neoplasia, e.g. transitional cell carcinoma, urethritis, calculi or foreign bodies
- *Other*: anticoagulants, urinary tract instrumentation, clotting abnormalities, trauma to the urinary tract, right-sided heart failure or renal vein thrombosis
- *Rare*: strenuous exercise, bacterial endocarditis or embolism

In this case the most likely diagnosis is a transitional carcinoma of the bladder. When taking the history it is important to elicit the following:

- *macro*scopic or *micro*scopic; duration of haematuria
- *age*: cancers are more common with increasing age
- *sex*: females more likely to have urinary tract infections
- *location*: during micturition was the haematuria always present (indicative of renal, ureteric or bladder pathology) or was it only present initially (suggestive of anterior urethral pathology) or present at the end of the stream (posterior urethra, bladder neck)?
- *pain*: more often associated with infection/inflammation/calculi, whereas malignancy tends to be painless
- associated lower urinary tract symptoms (irritative versus obstructive), which will be helpful in determining aetiology
- history of trauma
- travel abroad, e.g. swimming in lakes is Africa and Egypt and the risks of schistosomiasis
- previous urological surgery/history
- medication, e.g. anticoagulants
- family history
- occupational history, e.g. rubber/dye occupational hazards are risk factors for developing transitional carcinoma of the bladder due to exposure of chemicals such as β-naphthalene
- smoking status: increased risk, particularly of bladder cancer
- general status, e.g. weight loss, reduced appetite.

The patient should be resuscitated with intravenous fluids and a blood crossmatch taken. The INR of 2.2 is in the therapeutic range for her atrial fibrillation, but is unlikely to be the sole cause of her bleeding. Anticoagulation can often unmask other pathology in the urinary tract. Blood clots can cause urethral obstruction so a three-way catheter should be inserted and the bladder initially washed. The irrigation is continued until the haematuria begins to settle. The haemoglobin should be monitored and the patient transfused as necessary. A midstream urine should be sent for culture and antibiotic sensitivities. Urine cytology should also be sent to detect the presence of abnormal cells in the urine (once the haematuria has settled and the irrigation has stopped). The patient will require a urinary tract ultrasound to image the upper tracts and a flexible cystoscopy when the urine is clear. If these two last tests are negative, an intravenous urogram should be organized to exclude ureteric pathology.

KEY POINTS

- Patients with frank haematuria and persistent microscopic haematuria need investigating with cytoscopy and upper tract imaging.
- Patients on oral anticoagulation who develop haematuria still require investigation.

CASE 63: DIFFICULTY PASSING URINE

History

An 81-year-old man presents to the emergency department complaining of difficulty in passing urine. On questioning, he reports a worsening urinary stream over the last 6 months, together with increased nocturia. There is a recent history of bedwetting. He has no pain. He opens his bowels 3–4 times a week and his last bowel motion was 2 days ago. He is on insulin for type 1 diabetes. He also takes aspirin 75 mg od and simvastatin 20 mg od. He lives alone and mobilizes well with a walking stick. He is a non-smoker and has the occasional whisky at night to help him sleep.

Examination

On examination of the abdomen, there is a palpable suprapubic mass, which is non-tender and dull to percussion. The rest of the abdomen and genitalia are unremarkable. Digital rectal examination reveals an enlarged smooth-feeling prostate gland.

INVESTIGATIONS

		Normal
Sodium	134 mmol/L	135–145 mmol/L
Potassium	5.1 mmol/L	3.5–5.0 mmol/L
Urea	20.2 mmol/L	2.5–6.7 mmmol/L
Creatinine	334 μmol/L	44–80 μmol/L

Questions

- What is the diagnosis?
- Why does he recently complain of bedwetting?
- How should this patient be managed?
- What features on digital rectal examination would make you suspicious of prostate cancer?

ANSWER 63

This patient has chronic urinary retention secondary to an enlarged prostate. Acute and chronic retention are usually differentiated by the presence or absence of pain. Acute retention is painful, unlike chronic retention, when the bladder accommodates the increase in volume over time. A recent history of bedwetting is associated with a picture of chronic retention with overflow incontinence which usually occurs at night.

A urethral catheter should be inserted and the colour of the urine and residual volume noted and recorded in the notes. In cases of chronic retention the residual is often high (>2 L). The urine output should be monitored, as the patient may develop a diuresis. If the urine output is greater than 250 mL/h, intravenous fluid replacement in the form of 0.9 per cent normal saline is necessary to avoid hypovolaemia. The urine should be dipstick tested and sent for microscopy and culture. If positive for infection, antibiotics should be started. His renal function needs to be monitored to assess a response to treatment, and if not improving early consultation with the renal physicians is recommended. Constipation or urinary tract infection can compound the problem and they need to be treated accordingly. Often the patient has a history of lower urinary tract symptoms, which in this case are both obstructive and irritative in nature.

A digital rectal examination should be performed for patients in retention, noting the following points:

- external appearance of the anal orifice
- rectal masses
- consistency of the prostate
- presence of a median sulcus
- presence of nodules within the prostate
- fixity of the prostate gland
- estimated size of the prostate gland
- anal tone.

Features that suggest carcinoma of the prostate include hard gland, loss of normal contour (craggy prostate), loss of the midline sulcus, palpable nodule and a fixed gland. In cases of benign prostatic hyperplasia, the prostate feels enlarged and smooth as in this case.

KEY POINTS

- Acute retention is differentiated from chronic retention by the presence of pain.
- Precipitating factors, e.g. constipation, urinary tract infection, excessive alcohol, need to be screened for in the history.

CASE 64: TESTICULAR LUMP

History

A 31-year-old male stockbroker presents with a lump in his right testicle. He tells you it is uncomfortable while walking, and describes a dragging sensation. He also complains of generally feeling 'run down' but puts this down to stress at work, and has an irritable cough. He is a smoker of 20 cigarettes a day.

Examination

On examination a 3 cm palpable lump is felt on the inferior aspect of the right testicle. The rest of the testis and epididymis can be felt separately, and the mass does not transilluminate. It is not particularly tender to palpation. Abdominal examination is unremarkable.

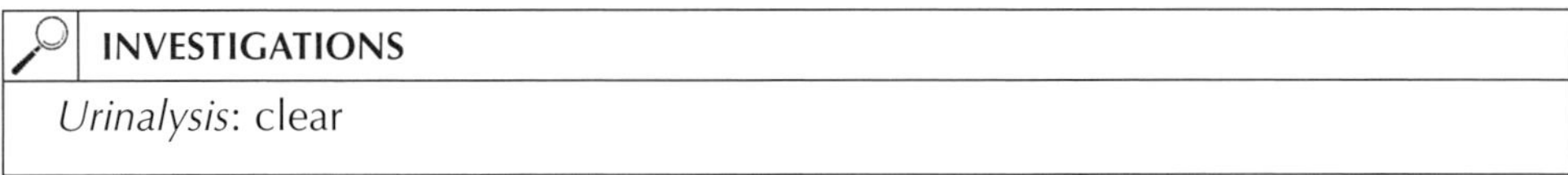

INVESTIGATIONS

Urinalysis: clear

Questions

- What is the likely diagnosis?
- What investigations are necessary?
- How do you differentiate between the different scrotal swellings?

ANSWER 64

The likely diagnosis is a testicular tumour. Ninety per cent of testicular tumours are germ cell tumours and are subdivided into seminomas and non-seminomatous germ cell tumours (NSGCT).

! Risk factors

- Age: common between 20 and 40 years
- Cryptorchidism
- Race: more common in Caucasians
- Previous testicular tumour
- Family history
- Klinefelter's syndrome

The patient's complaint of a cough should be taken seriously, as metastases to the lungs are possible with testicular tumours. A complete physical examination of the patient should be performed as there is potential for secondary deposits in the chest and brain. Lymphatic spread is to para-aortic lymph nodes in the abdomen rather than inguinal nodes in the groin, which only occur if the tumour erodes and involves the scrotal skin.

The diagnosis is confirmed with a scrotal ultrasound and serum tumour markers. Alpha-fetoprotein is elevated in NSGCT. The beta subunit of chorionic gonadotrophin (β-HCG) is elevated in NSGCT and in approximately 20 per cent of seminomas. Lactate dehydrogenase can be elevated in metastatic or bulky disease. All these markers are useful in monitoring disease progression and recurrence following various treatments. A computerized tomography scan of the chest and abdomen is required for staging purposes.

When examining a lump in the scrotum it is important to determine whether you can get above the swelling. If you cannot get above the swelling then it may be a hernia. You should then ask yourself the following questions:

- can the testis and epididymis be felt?
- does the swelling transilluminate?
- is the swelling tender?
- *Lump not confined to the scrotum* (cannot get above the lump):
  - inguino-scrotal hernia: unable to get above swelling, cough impulse, does not transilluminate, can feel testis separately
  - infantile communicating hydrocoele: unable to get above swelling, no cough impulse, transilluminates, cannot feel testis separately
- *Lump confined to the scrotum* (can get above the lump):
  - vaginal hydrocoele: testis and epididymis not felt easily, swelling transilluminates
  - haematocoele, syphilitic gumma, tumour: testis not readily identifiable, lump does not transilluminate
  - epididymal cyst: lump arising from epididymis which is felt and easily definable, swelling transilluminates
  - infection, e.g. epididymo-orchitis, TB or tumour: testis identifiable does not transilluminate

Acute inflammatory conditions such as epididymo-orchitis and acute haematocoele are associated with severe tenderness and erythema of the overlying skin.

KEY POINT

- Systematic examination is crucial in differentiating the causes of a scrotal swelling.

ORTHOPAEDIC

CASE 65: A FALL ONTO THE OUTSTRETCHED HAND

History

A 76-year-old woman is brought to the emergency department having fallen on the ice. She remembers slipping over and stretching out her right hand in order to 'save her fall'. She describes significant pain around her right wrist. Fortunately, her only other injury is a minor graze on her forehead. She says she has previously had a heart attack in her 60s. She takes atenolol, ramipril, simvastatin and aspirin. She also has a history of essential hypertension and she had a hysterectomy for menorrhagia when she was 40 years old. She is the sole carer for her husband who suffered a stoke 2 years ago and is bed-bound. She is anxious to get back home to look after him.

Examination

Her vital observations are stable. She has an obvious deformity of her right wrist. There is already bruising evident. There is no distal neurovascular deficit.

INVESTIGATIONS

Anterior-posterior and lateral X-rays of her wrist have been performed and are shown in Fig. 65.1.

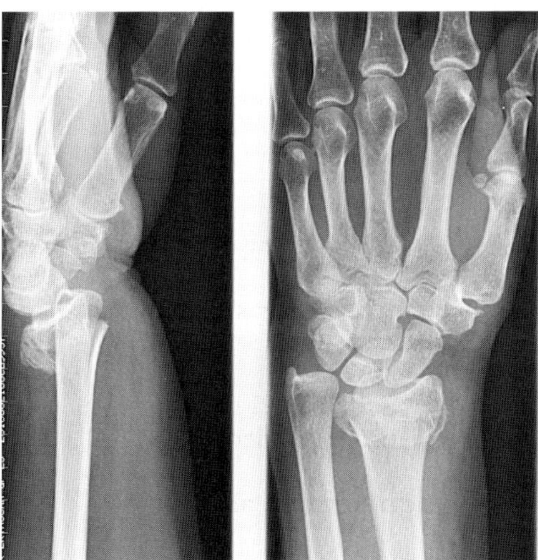

Figure 65.1 Plain X-rays of the right wrist.

Questions

- What injury has this woman sustained?
- How should it be managed?
- Are there any other considerations before this woman is sent home?

ANSWER 65

This woman has sustained a Colles' fracture. This term is often applied to any distal radial fracture. The correct definition of this injury comes from Abraham Colles in 1814, who originally described a low-energy extra-articular fracture of the distal radius occurring in elderly individuals. The typical mechanism of injury has been given in this scenario, which is a fall on the outstretched hand resulting in forced extension at the wrist. The distal fragment is dorsally angulated and displaced, giving a 'dinner-fork deformity' appearance (arrows in Fig. 65.2).

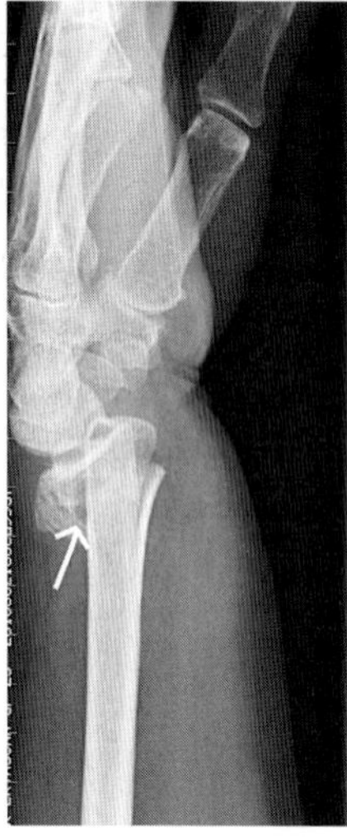
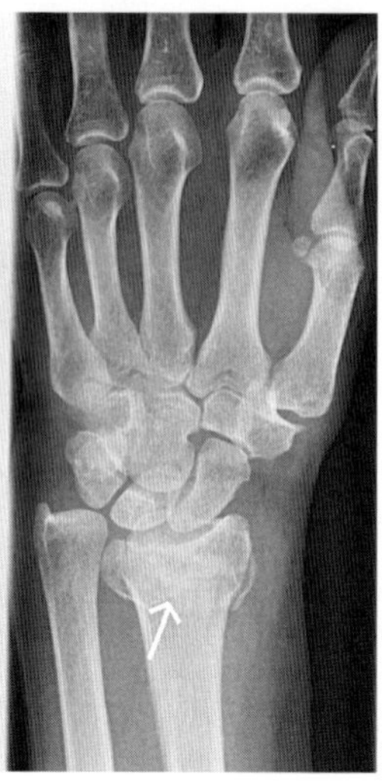

Figure 65.2 Colles' fracture (anterior-posterior and lateral).

It is important as with all injuries to assess the distal neurovascular status. In this injury it is not uncommon to develop symptoms associated with compression of the median nerve.

A Colles' fracture can usually be managed by closed reduction and immobilization. A number of techniques have been described. Adequate analgesia can be provided locally with lidocaine injected into the fracture site, a so-called haematoma block, or regional anaesthesia is used. The latter is thought to provide better pain control as well as allowing more accurate fracture reduction and a better functional outcome.

To achieve fracture reduction the distal fragment is further dorsally angulated in order to disengage it from the fracture site. Longitudinal traction is then applied while trying to manipulate that fragment in a distal and volar direction, thereby restoring the normal position and length to the radius. A backslab is applied with the wrist held in slight flexion and ulnar deviation. X-rays should be performed to check that there has been an adequate fracture reduction. The patient should be brought back to the fracture clinic in a few days in order to complete the cast and check that the fracture has not slipped out of position.

This case also illustrates the secondary consequences of significantly injuring a limb. It is unlikely that this woman will be able to cope at home, looking after her incapacitated husband. Most hospitals and general practitioners have access to a 'rapid response team', which is ideally suited to provide extra community-based social, nursing and physiotherapy support on a short-term basis.

KEY POINT

- In all fractures the distal neurological and vascular status should be assessed.

CASE 66: CHRONIC KNEE PAIN

History

A 67-year-old woman presents to her general practitioner with a history of progressive pain affecting her left knee. Over the last 3 months she has required increasing amounts of painkillers to control the pain. The pain gets worse throughout the day particularly if she has been very active, and it often keeps her awake at night. There is no history of significant trauma and she denies any other joint symptoms. She is otherwise fit and does not take any regular medication other than analgesics.

Examination

Examination of her left knee demonstrates a moderate swelling with a palpable effusion. The medial joint line is tender. The passive range of movement, which is painful, is restricted to an arc of 75°, and crepitus is felt throughout. The knee is intrinsically stable. The hip and ankle joints both have a full pain-free range of movement, and examination of her back is normal.

INVESTIGATIONS

An X-ray of the knee is taken, and is shown in Fig. 66.1.

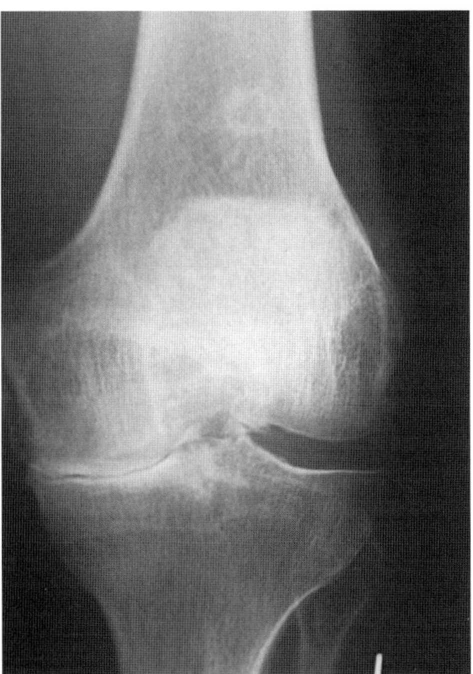

Figure 66.1 Plain X-ray of the left knee.

Questions

- What is the diagnosis?
- What are the typical X-ray findings in this condition?
- Which are the treatment options?

ANSWER 66

The anterior-posterior (AP) radiograph of the left knee demonstrates osteoarthritis (Fig. 66.2).

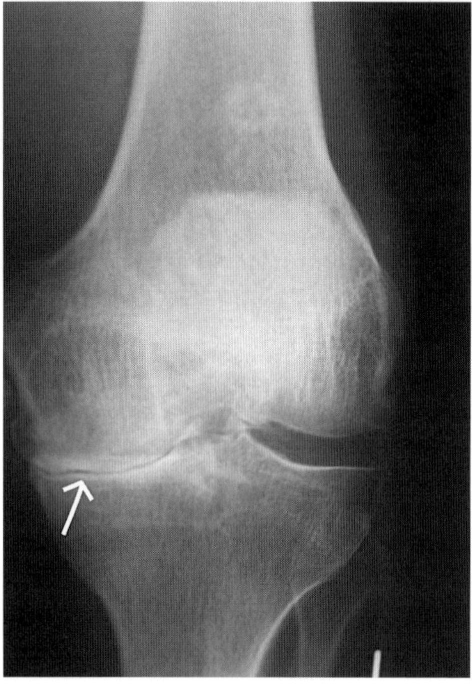

Figure 66.2 Osteoarthritis of the left knee (anterior-posterior).

The characteristic radiological features of osteoarthritis in *any* joint are:

- reduction in joint space
- osteophytes
- subchondral cyst formation
- periarticular sclerosis.

In this X-ray there is loss of the joint space on the medial side and periarticular sclerosis (arrow in Fig. 66.2).

Primary osteoarthritis is a common degenerative condition predominantly affecting the elderly population. The condition typically affects the weight-bearing joints, i.e. knee, hip, cervical and lumbar spine and ankle. The other common sites are the distal interphalangeal joints of the hands.

Radiological evidence of osteoarthritis is common, with 80 per cent of individuals over 80 years demonstrating some evidence of the condition. The symptoms of the disease do not, however, directly correlate with the radiological findings. A significant number of individuals remain symptom free despite radiographs showing extensive joint destruction. The commonest symptoms are pain, a reduction in mobility, and deformity of the affected joint. Diagnosis is made on a combination of clinical and radiological grounds. It is important when assessing the patient to examine the joints above and below as referred pain must be considered. Blood tests add little value if the history is typical.

Management is wide-ranging and crosses many disciplines. Surgical intervention should be considered if conservative measures fail and the condition significantly impairs the patient's quality of life.

- *Physiotherapy*: muscle strengthening exercises, walking aids
- *Occupational therapy*: hand rails, stair lifts, kitchen aids
- *Medical treatment* (non-invasive): simple analgesics, non-steroidal anti-inflammatory drugs
- *Medical treatment* (invasive): steroid joint injection, hyaluronan injections
- *Surgical intervention*: arthroscopy, osteotomies, arthroplasties

KEY POINTS

- Osteoarthritis primarily affects the weight-bearing joints.
- Management requires a multidisciplinary team approach.

CASE 67: SUDDEN CALF PAIN

History

A 31-year-old man attends the emergency department complaining of pain affecting his left calf. He was playing squash when he suddenly felt as though he had been hit on the back of the ankle. A loud snapping sound accompanied the pain.

Examination

Examination of the left foot and ankle reveals no obvious deformity. There is tenderness over the calf and posterior aspect of the ankle. There is a full passive range of movement of the foot, ankle and knee joints. There are normal foot pulses, and neurological examination is unremarkable.

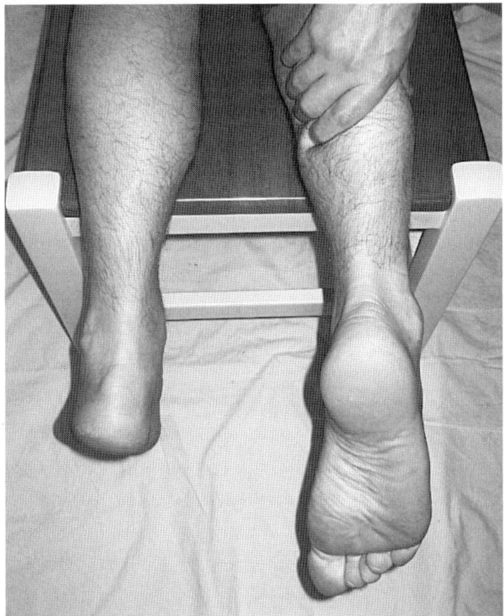

Figure 67.1

Questions

- What clinical test is being demonstrated on a normal leg in Fig. 67.1?
- What is the likely diagnosis in this patient?
- What investigation can be performed if the diagnosis is in question?

ANSWER 67

The clinical test that is being demonstrated is the 'Simmonds test'. It describes the absence of ankle plantar flexion when the calf is compressed. This picture demonstrates normal plantar flexion with calf compression on the right leg.

Failure of plantar flexion indicates that the patient has ruptured their Achilles tendon. The history of sudden pain affecting the calf during sporting activity is typical. Other examination findings may include a palpable gap in the Achilles tendon and an inability to actively plantar flex the ankle (i.e. the patient is unable to stand on 'tip toes'). The latter feature may be misleading, as the deep flexors of the foot can compensate for this movement.

An ultrasound scan can confirm a gap in the Achilles tendon when the diagnosis is in doubt. Serial ultrasound scans can also be used to assess healing of the tendon. There is debate as to the best way to treat this injury. Non-surgical management involves immobilizing the leg in a plaster of Paris cast, with the foot initially in full plantar flexion. While this avoids the risks of surgery, it delays functional rehabilitation and results in a greater risk of the tendon re-rupturing. The tendon can be repaired surgically, which is thought to result in a stronger tendon repair. This may be more appropriate for patients who require a greater level of sporting activity.

KEY POINTS

- Ultrasound can be used to detect damage to the Achilles tendon.
- Simmonds test is diagnostic of an Achilles tendon rupture.

CASE 68: LEFT KNEE INJURY

History

A 22-year-old woman is brought to the emergency department by ambulance. Her friend says that they had been out drinking and that she had fallen off a 4-foot wall landing directly on her left knee. Her knee swelled up immediately and she has not attempted to walk since the injury. She is normally fit and healthy. She takes the combined oral contraceptive pill, smokes 10–20 cigarettes a day and works in a supermarket.

Examination

Her observations are normal. There is no evidence of a head injury. Her left knee is diffusely swollen and there is evidence of bruising. The skin is intact. The medial and lateral joint lines are not tender. The patient is unable to actively extend the knee. The knee feels otherwise stable. The hip and ankle joints are unremarkable, and the pedal pulses and foot sensation are normal.

INVESTIGATIONS

Plain X-rays of the left knee are taken and are shown in Figs 68.1 and 68.2.

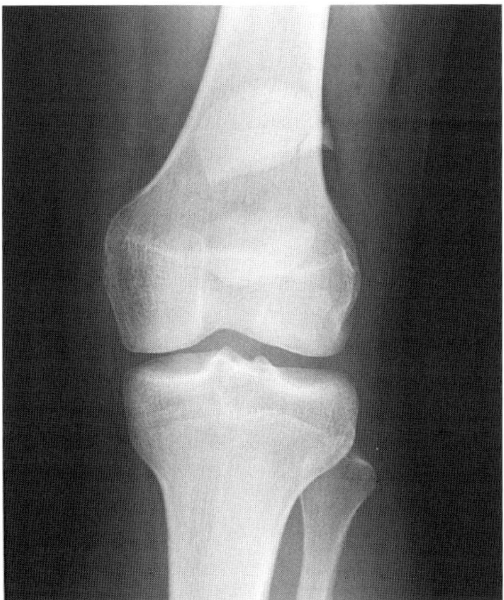

Figure 68.1 Plain X-ray of the left knee.

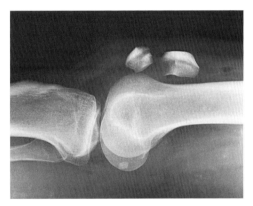

Figure 68.2 Plain X-ray of the left knee.

Questions

- What injury has this woman sustained?
- How should it be managed?

ANSWER 68

The X-rays show that the patient has a fractured patella (arrows in Figs 68.3 and 68.4).

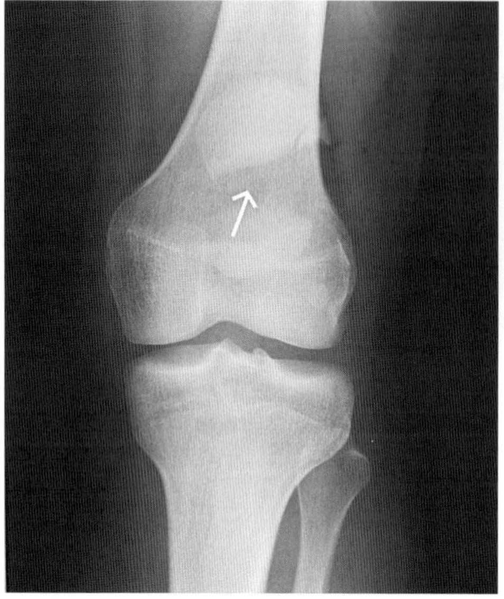

Figure 68.3 Patella fracture (anterior-posterior).

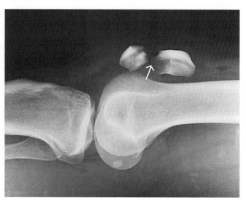

Figure 68.4 Patella fracture (lateral).

This type of fracture typically occurs with direct trauma to the knee. It is possible, however, to sustain a similar injury by an indirect mechanism, such as by vigorous jumping which leads to rapid flexion of the knee against a fully contracted quadriceps muscle. An indirect injury tends to result in less displacement and comminution of the fracture.

The patella is a large sesamoid bone. The upper border is connected to the quadriceps tendon and the lower pole is connected to the patella tendon, which inserts into the tibial tuberosity. In order to actively extend the knee, the whole unit must remain in continuity. It is, therefore, very important when examining knee injuries to ensure the extensor mechanism is intact by feeling for any palpable gap and by getting the patient to actively extend the knee.

Patella fractures can be managed conservatively or operatively. If the extensor mechanism is disrupted and/or there is a greater than 3 mm gap in the fracture site, surgical fixation is necessary. If the extensor mechanism is intact and there is a small gap in the fracture site, more common with the indirect injuries, then a cylinder plaster of Paris cast is more appropriate.

It is worth noting that a bipartite patella occurs in 1 per cent of the population, and it is not uncommon for patients to be misdiagnosed with a patella fracture. The diagnosis of a patella fracture is supported if there is a plausible mechanism of injury and the appropriate examination findings are present.

KEY POINT

- Bipartite patella occurs in 1 per cent of the population, and can be mistaken for a patella fracture.

CASE 69: RIGHT SHOULDER INJURY

History

A 23-year-old woman is brought to the emergency department having fallen over while on a dry ski slope. She is holding her right arm and is very reluctant to move her shoulder. She has previously had an appendicectomy and is known to have had mild attacks of asthma. She takes salbutamol and beclometasone regularly, and she is allergic to penicillin. She lives with her parents and works in the computer industry.

Examination

Her shoulder shows an obvious deformity and looks 'squared off', the arm is held in slight abduction and is externally rotated. Both active and passive movement of the shoulder cause pain. The radial pulse and capillary refill are normal.

INVESTIGATIONS

An X-ray of the shoulder is taken, and is shown in Fig. 69.1.

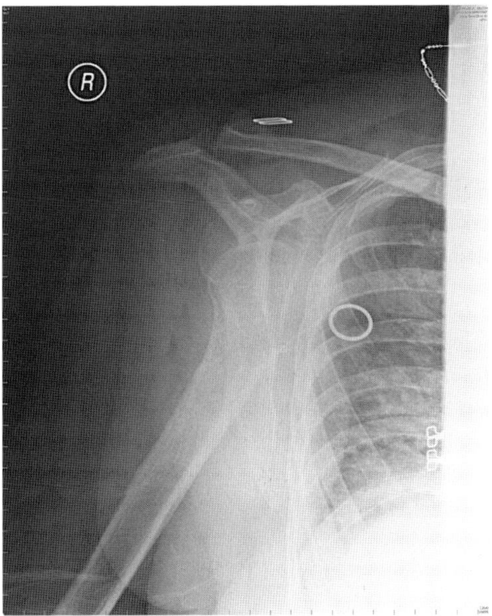

Figure 69.1 Plain X-ray of the right shoulder.

Questions

- What is the diagnosis?
- What are the other essential examination findings that have not been commented on?
- How should this injury be managed?

ANSWER 69

This patient has sustained an anterior dislocation of her right shoulder. Shoulder dislocations are the commonest joint dislocation, accounting for nearly half of all dislocations. The glenohumeral joint is a multi-axial 'ball and socket' joint and can, therefore, dislocate in any direction. However, in the majority of cases (90–98 per cent) the dislocation is anterior. Posterior dislocation is much less common and is typically secondary to either an epileptic fit or electric shock.

In order to confirm the diagnosis, radiographic assessment should be performed. The commonly used views are the anterior-posterior view in combination with either an axillary or scapular view. The important point is to examine the joint with two different views. The axillary view has the advantage of showing the glenoid cavity, which may pick up any associated fracture.

An assessment of both the distal vascular and neurological function must be made in any patient with a severe limb injury. The close relationship of the shoulder joint to the brachial plexus makes a nerve injury more likely. At particular risk are the radial and axillary nerves. The incidence of axillary nerve neuropraxias following anterior shoulder dislocation is quoted at up to 10 per cent. The axillary nerve supplies sensation to the lateral aspect of the upper arm, the 'regimental badge area'.

The majority of anterior shoulder dislocations can be replaced by closed reduction. The key to successful reduction is to ensure adequate analgesia. This will relax the shoulder musculature that is typically in spasm resisting any joint movement. After successful reduction, the patient should be able to touch the contralateral shoulder tip. The shoulder should be supported in a sling, with radiological confirmation of the reduction.

KEY POINTS

- A full neurological examination must be performed prior to reduction of any dislocated joint.
- The X-ray should be carefully examined for associated fractures.
- Adequate analgesia is crucial during reduction of the dislocation.

CASE 70: FALLS IN THE ELDERLY

History

A 78-year-old woman is brought in to the emergency department following a fall at home. She is complaining of severe pain affecting her left leg and groin, and has been unable to get up since the fall. On further questioning, the patient has been treated with steroids for polymyalgia rheumatica for the last 12 months and had sustained an injury of the right hip 5 years ago. Her only other medication is ramipril for essential hypertension. She lives independently in a three-bedroom, two-storey house and was widowed 4 years ago. She has a supportive son who normally visits her once a week.

Examination

The patient is now comfortable having been given intravenous morphine sulphate. Her left leg appears shorter than her right one and is externally rotated. She is unable to actively lift her leg, and any attempt to passively move it results in pain. Her pedal foot pulses and sensation are intact.

Questions

- What investigation is depicted in Fig. 70.1, and what does it show?
- What other relevant history would you wish to elicit?
- What would be the further management in this patient?
- Why is the social history particularly important in this patient?

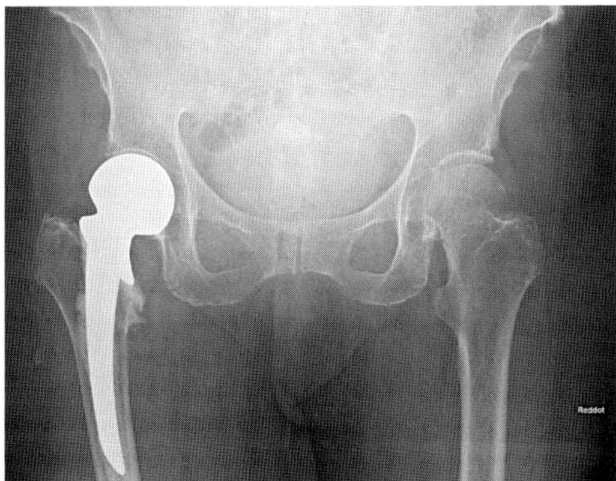

Figure 70.1 Plain X-ray of the pelvis.

ANSWER 70

This woman has sustained a (intracapsular) sub-capital neck of femur fracture. The X-ray also demonstrates a hip prosthesis on the right side, after a previous similar injury (arrow in Fig. 70.2).

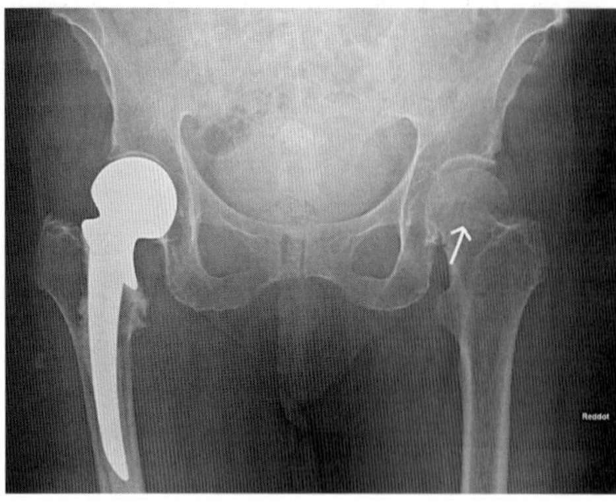

Figure 70.2 Fractured neck of femur on the left (anterior-posterior).

Fractured neck of the femur is a relatively common injury following a fall in the elderly population. The rate of hip fracture doubles every decade from the age of 50 years. There is a female preponderance of three to one. This woman is at particularly high risk because of her long-term steroid use. It is now a *British National Formulary* (*BNF*) recommendation that patients on long-term steroids should have concomitant treatment for the prevention of osteoporosis.

There are two different types of fractured neck of femur, intracapsular and extracapsular. Displaced fractures that are intracapsular disrupt the intra-osseous blood supply; the remaining blood supply comes from the retinacular vessels and from the artery of the ligamentum teres. This is usually not adequate to provide enough nutrition to allow fracture healing, leading to avascular necrosis of the femoral head. In this situation the fracture is not amenable to fixation; instead the head and proximal femoral neck are removed and replaced by a hemi-arthroplasty. Fractures that are extracapsular do not compromise the blood supply to the femoral head, so can be treated by fixation, i.e. a dynamic hip screw.

Irrespective of the fracture type, the initial management remains the same. It involves providing adequate analgesia, usually in the form of intravenous morphine. Intravenous fluid resuscitation is essential as these patients may well have been incapacitated for some time and will have sustained blood loss secondary to the fracture. Since these patients are likely to require an operation, they need a complete work-up for theatre. This will include blood tests (renal function, full blood count and group and save) and electrocardiogram and a chest X-ray if clinically indicated.

As part of the initial assessment it is important to take a comprehensive history, concentrating on of the mechanism of injury. It is incorrect to assume that all falls are mechanical; it is not uncommon to find the cause of the fall is actually due to a urinary or chest infection or even a silent myocardial infarction.

The patient's social history is also very important. The input of physiotherapists and occupational therapists is essential to ensure an adequate social care package is in place for discharge.

KEY POINTS

- Femoral neck fractures are classified as either intracapsular or extracapsular.
- Methods of surgical treatment depend on which type of fracture has been sustained.

CASE 71: LEFT HIP PAIN

History

A 67-year-old woman comes to see you in the orthopaedic outpatient clinic complaining of left groin pain. The pain has been present for the last 12 months and has become progressively worse. It initially responded to ibuprofen and paracetamol, but now the pain is keeping her awake at night. Over a similar time period there has been a reduction in mobility and she now uses a stick when going outside. There has been no history of injury and there are no neurological symptoms. She underwent a mastectomy for breast cancer 15 years ago. She takes tamoxifen and omeprazole.

Examination

She is overweight with a body mass index (BMI) of 31. She walks with an antalgic gait and has a positive Trendelenberg test. There is no gross deformity of the lower limbs and the real leg lengths are equal. There is a restriction of all her left hip movements, especially internal and external rotation. Her back and knee examinations are unremarkable. Her pedal pulses are palpable and the sensation in the leg is normal.

INVESTIGATIONS

An X-ray is taken and is shown in Fig. 71.1.

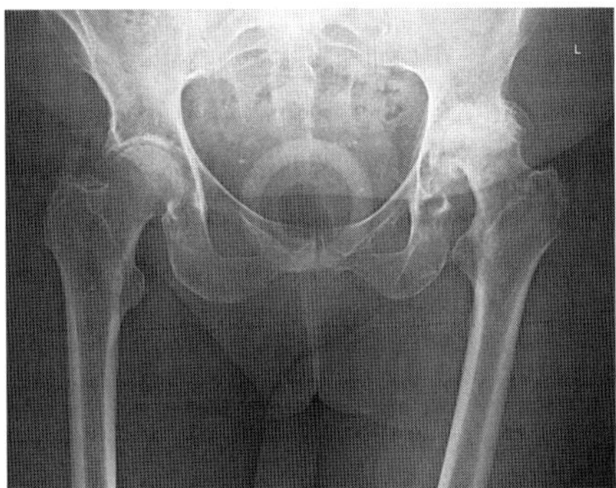

Figure 71.1 Plain X-ray of the pelvis.

Questions

- What do the X-rays show?
- What is a positive Trendelenberg test?
- What are the management options?

ANSWER 71

This woman has primary osteoarthritis of her left hip. There is a reduction in joint space and periarticular sclerosis seen in the left hip joint (Fig. 71.2).

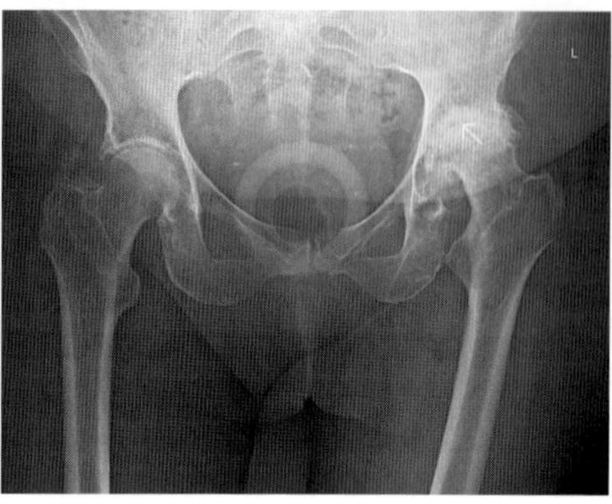

Figure 71.2 Osteoarthritis of the hip (anterior-posterior).

Primary osteoarthritis is by far the most common cause of joint degeneration. Less common is secondary osteoarthritis where there are a variety of different causative factors including developmental (congenital) dislocation of the hip, slipped upper femoral epiphysis, osteonecrosis and trauma.

Patients typically present with pain felt in the groin that may radiate to the knee, usually occurring after periods of activity. As the condition progresses, the pain is more constant and may cause sleep disturbance. Other symptoms may include stiffness, and limping.

The Trendelenberg test examines the strength and function of the hip abductor muscles. The examiner should perform the test by getting the patient to first stand on the 'good' leg and flex the other leg at the knee. This is repeated for the 'bad' leg. With normal function, the pelvis is held stable by the gluteus medius acting as an abductor in the supporting leg. A positive result is seen when the patient has a weak or a mechanically disadvantaged gluteus medius. This results in the pelvis 'sagging' down on the contralateral side. In this case when the patient stood on her *left* leg, the weakened gluteus medius on this side resulted in the *right* side of the pelvis dropping downwards.

A Trendelenberg gait demonstrates the same weak abductor mechanism. Normally when walking, the hip abductors are required to lift the pelvis and leg on the opposite side during the swing phase. If the abductors are not working, then the pelvis will tip downwards towards the lifted foot.

! Other frequent examination findings with osteoarthritis of the hip

- The affected leg is held adducted and in external rotation
- A positive Thomas' test: demonstrates a fixed flexion deformity
- Restriction of movements of the hip joint
- Normal knee and back examination

This woman's progressive symptoms and pain at night would suggest that she would benefit from a hip replacement.

KEY POINT

- The Trendelenberg test is used to determine the strength and function of the hip abductor muscles.

CASE 72: ASSESSMENT OF AN ANKLE INJURY

History

A 17-year-old boy is brought to the emergency department by his father, having fallen off his skateboard earlier on in the afternoon. He is complaining of ankle swelling and pain, and has been unable to fully weight-bear on his right leg. He is otherwise fit and healthy. He last ate a sandwich 7 h ago.

Examination

He has been assessed by the casualty officer, who reports that he warranted an X-ray based on the Ottawa rules.

INVESTIGATIONS

An X-ray is taken and is shown in Fig. 72.1.

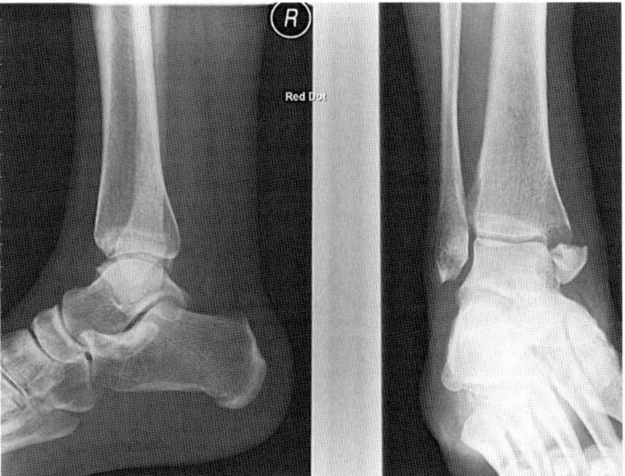

Figure 72.1 Plain X-rays of the ankle.

Questions

- What are the Ottawa rules?
- What does the X-ray show?
- What is the initial management?

ANSWER 72

The Ottawa rules have been developed to help clinicians make a decision as to whether an ankle (or mid-foot) injury warrants radiographic assessment:

- bone tenderness at the posterior edge or distal 6 cm or tip of the medial or lateral malleolus.
- bone tenderness at the base of the fifth metatarsal (for foot injuries)
- bone tenderness at the navicular bone (for foot injuries)
- unable *both* to weight-bear immediately after injury and walk four steps in the emergency department.

All suspected bony injuries should have X-rays taken in at least two different planes (normally anterior-posterior and lateral), to show whether there is a fracture. For the assessment of ankle injuries, mortise and lateral X-rays are taken. In this case the patient has sustained a fracture of the medial malleolus (arrows in Fig. 72.2).

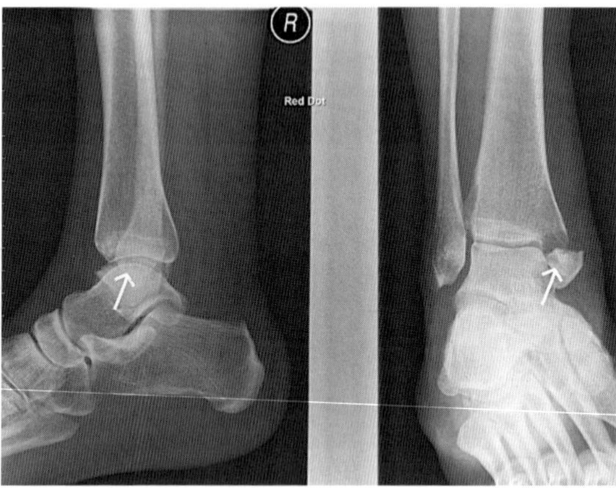

Figure 72.2 Fractured medial malleolus.

The initial principles of management of any closed fracture are the same. Having made the diagnosis of an ankle fracture, the fracture should be stabilized. Usually this involves applying a 'backslab' (a plaster of Paris cast that is a half-completed cylinder, which will mean that any resultant swelling is not restricted). It is important that the patient is provided with adequate analgesia; the act of stabilizing the fracture will reduce the fracture movement and so help with pain control. Stabilization will also allow the ankle and leg to be elevated to reduce the swelling. The next stages in the management are reduction of the fracture, and fixation. In this case the ankle will need operative fixation; this can potentially be performed quickly as the patient has fasted for over 6 h. However, if the ankle is too swollen and there is concern that the soft tissues will be compromised by the operation, then this will mean a delay by a matter of days.

KEY POINT

- The Ottawa rules can be used to determine if radiographical assessment of the ankle injury is required.

CASE 73: A PAINFUL AND SWOLLEN KNEE

History

A 63-year-old man with insulin-dependent diabetes mellitus attends the emergency department complaining of pain affecting his right knee. There is no history of significant trauma. On further questioning he had noticed that while gardening a few days previously he sustained a small graze to the skin in that area.

Examination

On examination he is febrile, (temperature 37.8°C), his blood pressure is 160/86 mmHg and his pulse rate is 96/min. Examination of his right knee reveals a red swollen joint that is tender. Attempting to move his knee both actively and passively results in severe pain. There is no abnormality to be found examining his right ankle or hip.

INVESTIGATIONS

		Normal
Haemoglobin	13.2 g/dL	11.5–16.0 g/dL
Mean cell volume	86 fL	76–96 fL
White cell count (WCC)	15.6×10^9/L	$4.0–11.0 \times 10^9$/L
Platelets	289×10^9/L	$150–400 \times 10^9$/L
Erythrocyte sedimentation rate	34 mm/h	10–20 mm/h
Sodium	135 mmol/L	135–145 mmol/L
Potassium	3.9 mmol/L	3.5–5.0 mmol/L
Urea	5.1 mmol/L	2.5–6.7 mmmol/L
Creatinine	78 μmol/L	44–80 μmol/L
C-reactive protein	145 mg/L	<5 mg/L

Questions

- What is the likely diagnosis?
- What should the initial management involve?

ANSWER 73

This man has a septic arthritis of the right knee. The localized redness and swelling can be associated with any inflammatory monoarthritis, but a septic arthritis is an important differential diagnosis suggested here by the history, examination findings and blood tests.

Septic arthritis can affect any joint. The most commonly affected joint is the knee (50 per cent of cases), followed by the hip (20 per cent), shoulder (8 per cent), ankle (7 per cent) and wrist (7 per cent). *Staphylococcus aureus* is the cause in the vast majority of cases of acute bacterial arthritis in adults. Streptococcal species, such as *Streptococcus viridans*, *Streptococcus pneumoniae*, and group B streptococci, account for 20 per cent of cases. Aerobic gram-negative rods are involved in 20–25 per cent of cases. Organisms may invade the joint by direct inoculation, spread from adjacent infected tissue, or via the bloodstream, which is the most common route. Following the initial stabilization of the patient (they may be unwell with signs of septic shock), the joint should be aspirated. The aspirated fluid should be sent to the laboratory for microscopy to look for pus cells and evidence of bacterial infection. The fluid should also be examined with polarizing microscopy to look for the presence of crystals. This is to exclude the differential diagnosis of crystal arthropathy (gout or pseudo-gout). Blood tests can be useful as they suggest the presence of infection (raised WCC and inflammatory markers). In addition, blood cultures should be sent as they may isolate a causative organism. Treatment of a septic joint should be prompt and effective. The joint should undergo a thorough washout followed by immobilization. High-dose empirical antibiotics should be administered intravenously until cultures and sensitivities are available. The major consequence of bacterial infection is damage to articular cartilage. This may be the result of the infective organism's pathological properties or the host's own immune response. Delay in the diagnosis and treatment will result in a poorly functioning joint.

KEY POINTS

- *Staphylococcus aureus* is the most common causative organism.
- Prompt treatment is required to prevent permanent damage to the joint.

CASE 74: PAINFUL HANDS

History

A 32-year-old woman, who is 36 weeks pregnant, visits her general practitioner complaining of pain affecting both hands. The pain has developed over the last 2 weeks, and is worse at night. She also describes a tingling sensation, particularly in the index and middle fingers. In order to relieve the pain the patient describes shaking her hands to get 'the circulation going'. There is no history of neck injury, and the pain only radiates as far as her elbows.

Examination

Examination of the patient's hands shows no obvious abnormality. The radial pulse and capillary return in both hands are normal.

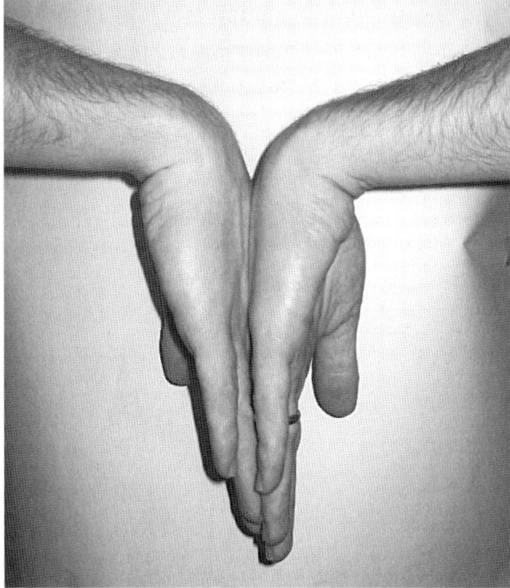

Figure 74.1

Questions

- What test is being demonstrated in Fig. 74.1?
- What additional clinical test can be performed to support the diagnosis?
- What is the cause of this patient's problem?
- How would it be best managed?

ANSWER 74

This woman has carpal tunnel syndrome. The condition is due to compression of the median nerve as it enters the hand through a 'tunnel' formed by the flexor retinaculum. Any reduction in this limited space produces pain and tingling along the course of the median nerve. The median nerve has both sensory and motor functions. It provides sensation to the volar aspect of the thumb, index and middle fingers, and half of the ring finger. This gives rise to the tingling sensation affecting only part of the hand. The motor supply is to the 'LOAF' muscles i.e. Lateral two Lumbricals, Opponens pollicis, Abductor pollicis brevis and Flexor pollicis brevis. If a patient has severe or long-standing carpal tunnel syndrome then they will complain of weakness and there may be signs of muscle wasting over the thenar eminence.

The tests used to support a diagnosis of carpal tunnel syndrome involve trying to further compress the median nerve in order to see if the patient's symptoms can be reproduced. The test shown in Fig. 74.1 is Phalen's test, which involves placing the wrist in maximal flexion for 1 min. An alternative test is Tinel's test, in which the examiner taps over the volar aspect of the wrist, in order to see if tingling/paraesthesia is produced in the median nerve distribution.

It is important, when examining a patient with suspected carpal tunnel syndrome, to carefully examine their neck, shoulder, and axilla. The symptoms of pain and paraesthesia suggest an entrapment neuropathy, and the source of the neurological compression may be proximal to the carpal tunnel, i.e. cervical disc prolapse, axilla lymph node mass compressing the brachial plexus. Where the diagnosis is uncertain, electrophysiological tests (electromyograms (EMGs)) can be performed to determine whether the median nerve is compressed and at which level.

! Causes of carpal tunnel syndrome

- Idiopathic
- Rheumatoid arthritis
- Wrist fracture
- Hypothyroidism
- Pregnancy
- Alcoholism
- Renal failure

Wrist splints may be the most appropriate treatment in this patient, while she is pregnant, as her symptoms are likely to improve after delivery. Alternative treatments include an injection of steroid around the carpal tunnel in order to reduce any swelling and associated inflammation. The definitive treatment is carpal tunnel release, which can be performed either endoscopically or as an open procedure. This patient's symptoms should improve after delivery of her child.

KEY POINT

- EMG studies can be used to confirm the diagnosis of carpal tunnel syndrome.

CASE 75: DISPROPORTIONATE PAIN

History

You are called to the orthopaedic ward to see a 42-year-old man who has been admitted earlier in the day following a motorcycle accident. He sustained a closed tibia and fibular fracture that has been treated in a backslab in anticipation of an operation tomorrow. The nursing staff report that he is complaining of pain despite receiving 20 mg of intravenous morphine. He is otherwise fit and healthy. He smokes 20 cigarettes a day and consumes on average 40 units of alcohol a week.

Examination

The patient is in obvious discomfort. His blood pressure is 160/90 mmHg and the pulse rate is 100/min. The affected leg is still wrapped in a crepe bandage covering the backslab. The pedal pulses are accessible and are intact.

Questions

- What diagnosis must you consider?
- What bedside tests could be performed to confirm the diagnosis?
- What are the initial steps in the management of this condition?

ANSWER 75

This patient requires urgent assessment, as he may have developed a compartment syndrome.

Within the limbs there are a number of myofascial compartments. These consist of muscles contained within a relatively fixed-volume structure, bounded by fascial layers and bone. After trauma the pressure in the myofascial compartment increases. This pressure may exceed the venous capillary pressure, resulting in a loss of venous outflow from the compartment. The failure to clear metabolites also leads to the accumulation of fluid as a result of osmosis. If left untreated, the pressure will eventually exceed arterial pressure, leading to significant tissue ischaemia. The damage is irreversible after 4–6 h.

Tibial fractures are the commonest cause of an acute compartment syndrome, which is thought to complicate up to 20 per cent of these injuries. The clue in this patient is the fact that he is still in significant pain despite intravenous opiate analgesia. The classical description of 'pain out of proportion to the injury' may be difficult to determine if the clinician is inexperienced. Passive stretching of the muscles in the affected compartment is a very useful bedside test. In this case, if passive extension of the toes elicits pain, then this would indicate increased pressure in the posterior compartment of the leg. The compartment pressures can also be measured directly using a slit catheter.

The limb should be fully exposed, as despite the fact that a backslab is not a complete cast, the bandages may still be responsible for causing occlusion. The definitive treatment is a fasciotomy to decompress the relevant myofascial compartments.

KEY POINT

- Suspected compartment syndrome should be dealt with promptly to avoid permanent muscle damage.

CASE 76: SPORTING KNEE DEFORMITY

History

A 16-year-old girl is brought to the emergency department by ambulance complaining of left-knee pain. She has been performing gymnastics at school and remembers twisting and then developing a severe pain around her knee. Her past medical history is unremarkable. She is allergic to penicillin. Her mum reports that both the patient and her sister are 'double jointed'.

Examination

She is holding her swollen left knee in a flexed position. There is an obvious deformity with a prominent bulge on the lateral aspect of the knee. She is very reluctant to move the knee actively. The distal neurovascular status is normal.

Questions

- What is the diagnosis?
- What manoeuvre can be performed to improve her pain and rectify the deformity?
- What should be the further management of the injury?

ANSWER 76

The patient has dislocated her patella. The injury is most common in adolescent females and in patients with joint laxity. One can also have an anatomical predisposition to dislocation: a relatively small lateral femoral condyle, genu valgum ('knock-knees'), patella alta (high-riding patella) or quadriceps weakness.

The examination findings of a flexed swollen knee and a large bulge laterally (dislocation of the patella medially is rare) should prompt the clinician to make the diagnosis. An initial X-ray is unnecessary, as it is important relocate the dislocated patella as soon as possible. This is achieved by getting the patient to lie supine with the hip flexed. The knee should then be passively extended while medial pressure is applied to the patella.

Following relocation, plain radiography should be performed, usually an anterior-posterior, true lateral and a skyline view of the patella. Although the injury mainly involves disruption of the medial soft-tissue structures of the knee, there is a 5 per cent incidence of associated osteochondral fracture. Plain radiography also provides information as to whether there are any of the anatomical risk factors listed above.

As this is the first episode of traumatic lateral patellar dislocation, without any associated fracture, it should be treated conservatively. The knee should be immobilized in extension, to allow the medial patello-femoral ligament to heal. Physiotherapy is then essential to build up the muscle strength and increase the stability of the patello-femoral joint. Unfortunately, up to 50 per cent of patients will have recurrent episodes of patello-femoral instability, which will require surgical intervention.

KEY POINTS

- Patella dislocation is most common in adolescent females.
- Up to 50 per cent can have recurrent symptoms requiring surgical intervention.

CASE 77: FOOTBALLER'S KNEE

History

A 34-year-old builder presents to the emergency department having injured his left knee earlier that afternoon while playing football. He describes being tackled and feeling his knee twist inwards. Immediately after the injury his knee began to swell and he was unable to continue playing. He now has only limited movement of his knee and is unable to walk.

He is otherwise fit and healthy and does not take any regular medication. He has a wife and two children and smokes 20 cigarettes a day. His average alcohol intake is 34 units a week.

Examination

The left knee is held in approximately 30° of flexion. It is swollen and there is an obvious effusion. Palpation elicits localized tenderness along the medial tibio-femoral joint line. It is not possible to fully extend the knee either passively or actively. The ligamentous stability of the knee appears normal. Neurovascular examination of the limb is normal.

Questions

- What is the likely injury?
- What are the other causes of a haemarthrosis?
- How should this patient be managed?

ANSWER 77

This man has sustained a meniscal injury. Most knee injuries result in swelling which develops over hours rather than minutes. The history of immediate knee swelling suggests that there is a haemarthrosis. (This can be easily confirmed by aspirating a few millilitres of fluid from the joint using an aseptic no-touch technique).

! Causes of a haemarthrosis

- Anterior cruciate tear: in 75 per cent of cases
- Meniscal tear
- Fracture
- Spontaneous haemarthrosis: haemophilia

It is not uncommon to sustain a simultaneous cruciate and meniscal injury. In practice it is often difficult to assess the ligamentous stability in the acutely injured knee and make a definitive diagnosis on clinical examination alone. However, in this case the findings of a 'locked' knee, and the fact there was thought to be no ligamentous deficiency, suggest an isolated meniscal injury. The classical cause of an acutely 'locked' knee is a 'bucket-handle meniscal tear'. This refers to a longitudinal full-thickness tear of the meniscus. The flap which is created can flip into the joint on the other side of the femoral condyle, blocking full extension of the knee.

The blood supply of the meniscus is located at its periphery, the 'red zone'. The inner 'white' portion is avascular. The importance of this relates to the location of any meniscal tear; if confined to the red zone then there is the potential for repair and subsequent healing. In this scenario the patient should be taken to theatre for an arthroscopy. As well as allowing the knee to be 'unlocked', it will provide a definitive diagnosis, with the potential to repair the meniscal tear.

KEY POINTS

- A history of immediate knee swelling suggests a haemarthrosis.
- A locked knee can be caused by a bucket-handle meniscal tear.

CASE 78: PAINFUL LIMB IN SICKLE CELL DISEASE

History

A 15-year-old boy with known sickle cell disease, presents to the emergency department with pain in his right leg. The pain has been worsening over the last 4 days and he is now barely able to walk. He has an associated fever and lethargy. There is no reported history of trauma and he is taking prophylactic penicillin.

Examination

His temperature is 37.8°C and pulse rate 114/min. His oxygen saturations are 91 per cent on room air. He looks unwell and is in severe pain. There is no obvious abnormality of his right leg. He has significant tenderness over his right thigh. He has normal knee and hip movements. The neurovascular examination of his limb is unremarkable.

INVESTIGATIONS

		Normal
Haemoglobin	6.3 g/dL	11.5–16.0 g/dL
Mean cell volume	86 fL	76–96 fL
White cell count (WCC)	15.6×10^9/L	$4.0–11.0 \times 10^9$/L
Platelets	289×10^9/L	$150–400 \times 10^9$/L
Erythrocyte sedimentation rate (ESR)	89 mm/h	10–20 mm/h
Sodium	137 mmol/L	135–145 mmol/L
Potassium	3.9 mmol/L	3.5–5.0 mmol/L
Urea	9.1 mmol/L	2.5–6.7 mmmol/L
Creatinine	78 µmol/L	44–80 µmol/L
C-reactive protein (CRP)	137 mg/L	<5 mg/L

Questions

- What is the cause of his pain?
- How should this patient be managed acutely?
- What is the differential diagnosis in a patient with sickle cell disease?

ANSWER 78

Sickle cell anaemia is an autosomal recessive genetic disease that results from the substitution of valine for glutamic acid at position 6 of the beta-globin gene, leading to production of a defective form of haemoglobin, hemoglobin S (HbS). Deoxygenation of HbS leads to distortion of the red blood cell into the classic sickle shape. The sickle cells are much less deformable than normal red cells and can obstruct the microcirculation. This results in tissue hypoxia, which causes further sickling. Patients with a sickle cell crisis should be treated with high-flow oxygen, opioid analgesia and fluid resuscitation. If the precipitating factor is thought to be infective then intravenous antibiotics should be started.

! Causes of sickle cell crises

- Dehydration
- Bleeding
- Infection
- Hypoxia
- Cold exposure
- Drug and alcohol use
- Pregnancy and stress

Limb and back pain are common presentations for sickle cell sufferers. Osteomyelitis should be considered as a differential diagnosis, although bone infarction secondary to a sickle crisis is 50 times more common. The two conditions have a similar presentation with common features:

- pain
- fever
- tenderness
- inflammation
- raised inflammatory markers (CRP, ESR and WCC).

Radiographs are of limited use in the acute phase of osteomyelitis, as bone destruction and periosteal reaction do not become evident until at least 10 days. A more sensitive investigation is a technetium bone scan which is reported to detect signs of osteomyelitis after 3 days. Magnetic resonance imaging is also useful in helping to identify abscesses, sequestra and sinus tracts. A fine-needle bone aspirate provides a definitive diagnosis and can isolate the causative organism. The most common organism is *Staphylococcus aureus*. In sickle cell sufferers this remains the likely organism, but *Salmonella* and *Enterobacter* are also commonly cultured.

KEY POINTS

- Radiographical evidence of osteomyelitis may not be present during the first 10 days.
- A sickle cell crisis should be initially treated with analgesia, oxygen and fluids.

CASE 79: NECK INJURIES

History

A 27-year-old man is brought in to the emergency department by ambulance. He had been playing prop forward in a rugby match when the scrum suddenly collapsed. After the scrum had been cleared, he was found conscious on the ground unable to move his arms or legs. He has no significant past medical history. He does not smoke or drink alcohol. He normally works as a bank manager.

Examination

The patient is alert and talking. He is lying supine on a spinal board with his neck immobilized in a hard collar. The chest is clear with good breath sounds throughout both lungs. His blood pressure is 92/42 mmHg and the pulse rate is 62/min. He has warm peripheries and his abdomen is soft. Examination of his neurological system confirms complete flaccidity of his arms and legs. He has no sensation from the shoulders downwards, and absent reflexes.

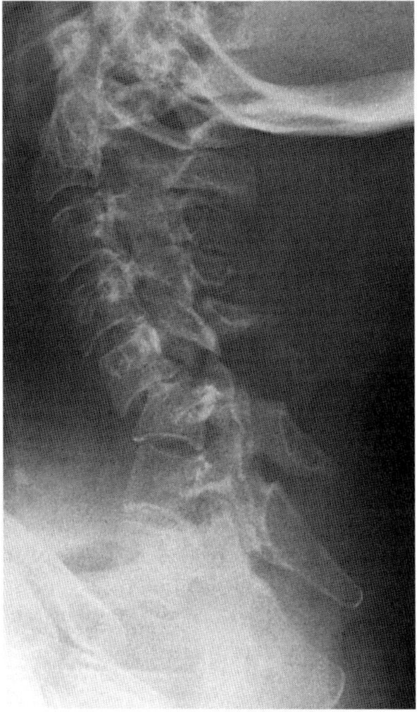

Figure 79.1 Lateral view of the cervical spine.

Questions

- What investigation is shown?
- What is the diagnosis?
- What is the explanation for the patient's vital signs?

ANSWER 79

This man has sustained a cervical spine fracture and associated spinal cord injury. The investigation shown is a lateral C-spine X-ray and demonstrates a fracture dislocation at the level of C5/C6 (arrow in Fig. 79.2).

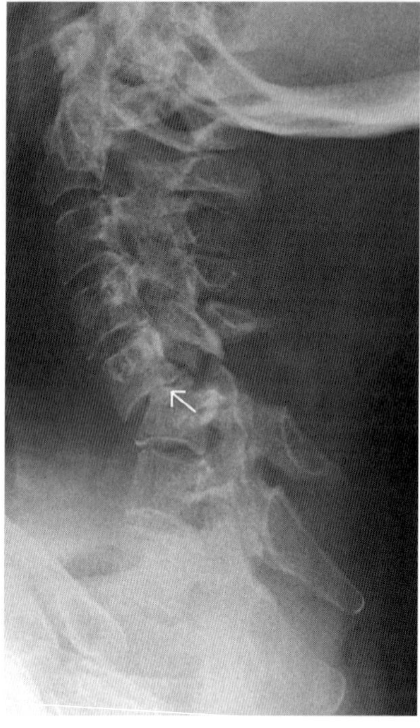

Figure 79.2 Fracture dislocation at the level of C5/C6 (arrow).

In addition this patient is exhibiting signs of neurogenic spinal shock. This is caused by vasomotor instability and loss of sympathetic tone as a result of spinal cord damage. He is hypotensive and has a paradoxical bradycardia, which should not be confused with hypovolaemic shock where there is hypotension and tachycardia.

A 'concussive' type of injury to the cord can cause a transient flaccid paralysis, 'spinal shock', which may recover over 24–72 h but can take weeks. Any recovery in segmental reflexes has a significant effect on long-term prognosis, and the term 'incomplete spinal cord injury' applies. If there is no return in motor or sensory function below the level of the injury then this is a 'complete' injury and no further recovery can be expected.

Neck injuries are a common presentation to the emergency department. They should all be taken seriously and appropriately assessed. There are a number of guidelines (Canadian C-Spine Rules and National Emergency X-Radiography Utilization Group – NEXUS) that have been drawn up to help clinicians rule out a significant injury. The NEXUS rules suggest that to be able to 'clear' the cervical spine clinically, the following criteria must be met:

- a normal conscious level (Glasgow Coma Score 15)
- no evidence of intoxication
- no distracting injury
- no posterior midline cervical spine tenderness
- no focal neurological deficit.

When investigating a patient with a suspected C-spine injury, the first-line investigation is a plain radiograph of the cervical spine. As part of the Advanced Trauma and Life

Support (ATLS) management protocol, a lateral view of the cervical spine is performed. This will pick up 85 per cent of cervical spine injuries and so is a useful as a screening test. Anterior-posterior and odenotoid peg views should also be obtained.

Plain radiography is, however, not infallible and where there is still a clinical suspicion of a cervical spine injury then a computerized tomography (CT) scan should be performed.

KEY POINTS

- All suspected C-spine injuries should be immobilized before clinical assessment, followed by radiological investigation if indicated.
- Plain radiographs do not exclude all fractures; if there is doubt a CT should be obtained.

CASE 80: A LIMPING CHILD

History

A 13-year-old boy presents to his general practitioner with an 8-week history of an ache in the left thigh. Over the last few days this has got worse and now he is complaining of groin pain and has developed a pronounced limp. He is unsure, but his worsening symptoms may have coincided with a fall while playing football. He is feeling well and reports no back or neurological symptoms. His past medical history is unremarkable and he takes no regular medication.

Examination

His pulse and blood pressure are within the normal range and he is afebrile. He is overweight and has a body mass index of 33. His abdominal examination is normal and there are no detectable abnormalities of the back or left knee. His left leg is held in slight external rotation. There is a restriction in abduction and internal rotation. When the hip is flexed the leg is forced into external rotation. There is no distal neurovascular deficit.

INVESTIGATIONS

An X-ray is taken and is shown in Fig. 80.1.

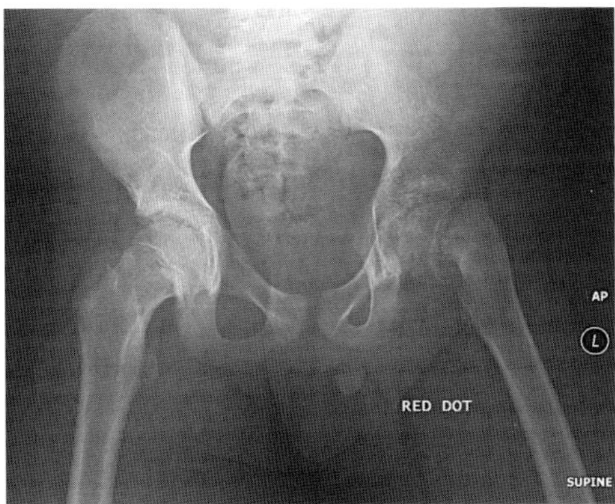

Figure 80.1 Plain X-ray of the pelvis.

Questions

- What is the diagnosis?
- What further plain X-rays should be requested?
- What are the other causes of a 'limping child'?

ANSWER 80

This boy has a (acute-on-chronic) slipped capital femoral epiphysis (arrow in Fig. 80.2).

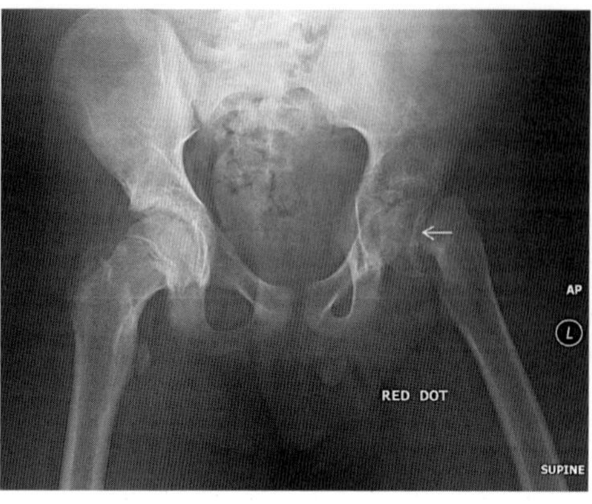

Figure 80.2 Slipped femoral epiphysis of the left hip.

This refers to a weakening or fracture of the proximal femoral epiphyseal growth plate. Continued shear stresses on the hip cause the epiphysis to move posteriorly and medially. This condition has a peak presentation in adolescent boys. There are a number of risk factors including obesity, hypothyroidism and renal failure.

There are three different types described:

- *acute slip*: normally secondary to significant trauma
- *chronic slip*: the commonest (60 per cent) presentation with symptoms >3 weeks
- *acute-on-chronic*: duration of symptoms >3weeks with sudden deterioration.

This scenario is also an excellent example of the orthopaedic mantra of examining the 'joint above and below' the suspected origin of the pathology. Up to half of the patients with a chronic slipped capital femoral epiphysis present with thigh or knee pain. In this case one of the important clues in the examination is the finding of obligatory external rotation when the hip is flexed.

The anterior-posterior X-ray demonstrates Trethowan's sign. When a line (Klein line) is drawn along the superior surface of the neck, it should pass through part of the femoral head. If the line remains superior to the femoral head then this is termed Trethowan's sign. A frog-lateral view of the hip is normally requested to further aid diagnosis, although caution should be applied in acute presentations as this can worsen the slip. It is also worth noting that when a patient is diagnosed with a slipped capital femoral epiphysis, an X-ray of the opposite hip should be performed as a bilateral presentation occurs in one-third of patients.

At any age, a limp in a child should always be taken seriously. General points to note are: if the child is febrile or unwell then the diagnosis of a septic arthritis or osteomyelitis should be considered. In the well child, trauma and neoplasia can occur in all age groups. The limping infant should make the clinician think of a developmental hip dysplasia, whereas in the 4–10-year age range, one should think of Perthes' disease.

KEY POINT

- The joints above and below the presumed source of the pain should always be examined.

CASE 81: ORTHOPAEDIC TRAUMA

History

A 23-year-old man is brought into the emergency department by ambulance after coming off his motorcycle. He was travelling at approximately 45 mph and hit a stationary car. A trauma call is made and you are the orthopaedic member of the trauma team. There is no other history available and he is in significant pain.

Examination

The patient's pulse is 100/min, blood pressure is 142/88 mmHg and his oxygen saturations are 97 per cent on room air. His Glasgow Coma Score has remained at 15 out of 15. He is strapped onto a spinal board. The trauma team has completed the initial assessment of the patient. The primary survey has been completed and there is no significant chest, abdominal or pelvic injury.

Examining the left leg, there is an obvious deformity. His shin is angulated at 45°. There is a 3 cm-diameter wound, which has bone protruding through it. The pedal pulses are palpable. The distal sensation is intact.

INVESTIGATIONS

An X-ray is taken and is shown in Fig. 81.1.

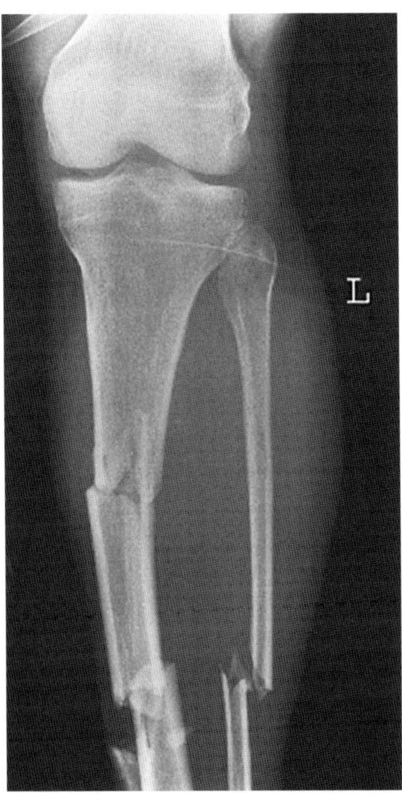

Figure 81.1 Plain X-ray of the left leg.

Questions

- What are the principles of initial assessment of a trauma patient?
- What is involved in a trauma X-ray series?
- What is the initial management for this patient's leg injury?

ANSWER 81

Most emergency departments have a protocol to deal with patients involved in significant trauma, which is based around the Advanced Trauma and Life Support (ATLS) guidelines. This involves a primary survey concerned with diagnosing and treating life-threatening injuries quickly and effectively. The assessment follows an *'ABCDE' approach:*

- *A*: airway with cervical spine protection
- *B*: breathing and ventilation
- *C*: circulation with haemorrhage control
- *D*: disability – neurological status
- *E*: exposure/environmental control.

The trauma series of X-rays are typically comprised of an anterior-posterior (AP) chest X-ray, an AP pelvis X-ray and a lateral C-spine X-ray. This combination of X-rays is aimed at picking up major injuries such as a haemothorax or pelvic fracture.

When the primary survey has been completed and resuscitation has been commenced, a secondary survey is performed. This is a 'head to toe' examination to determine any other injuries.

In this case the patient has sustained an 'open' or 'compound' tibial fracture. While this is not life-threatening, it is important it is dealt with promptly. The normal principles when dealing with any fracture still apply, i.e. analgesia, stabilization, elevation, reduction and fixation. The wound should be photographed and covered with gauze soaked in an antiseptic solution. This avoids the necessity of repeated re-examinations which would increase the risk of infection before reaching the operating theatre. Intravenous broad-spectrum antibiotics should be commenced as soon as possible e.g. cefuroxime and metronidazole. Similarly tetanus prophylaxis should be considered and given if necessary. Providing the patient is otherwise stable, they should be taken to theatre for wound debridement and irrigation.

KEY POINT

- The ATLS protocol should be followed even in the presence of obvious limb deformity, to ensure a potentially life-threatening injury is not missed.

EAR, NOSE AND THROAT

CASE 82: SORE THROAT

History

A 28-year-old man arrives at the emergency department complaining of a sore throat. The pain has been increasing over the last few days and he is now finding it difficult to open his mouth. He has stopped eating and is only tolerating small amounts of fluid. Two days ago he saw his general practitioner who prescribed him some oral antibiotics and analgesia for a mild tonsillitis. He suffers with asthma.

Examination

He appears uncomfortable and has difficulty in speaking as a result of his pain. His blood pressure is stable, but his temperature is 39.0°C and his pulse rate is 115/min. His oxygen saturation is 98 per cent on room air. Oral examination, with a tongue depressor, reveals a unilateral left-sided tonsillar swelling with a diffuse oedematous 'bulge' superior and lateral to the tonsil. As a result the uvula is deviated to the contralateral side. The left tonsil has some exudate on its surface. There is a palpable jugulo-digastric lymph node on the left. The rest of the examination is unremarkable.

INVESTIGATIONS

		Normal
Haemoglobin	14.8 g/dL	11.5–16.0 g/dL
White cell count	18.0 × 10^9/L	4.0–11.0 × 10^9/L
Platelets	301 × 10^9/L	150–400 × 10^9/L

Questions

- What is the diagnosis?
- What is the initial management?
- What is the differential diagnosis?

ANSWER 82

The patient has a left-sided quinsy or peritonsillar abscess. This occurs between the palatine tonsil and the pharyngeal muscles. It develops from an untreated or ineffectively treated acute exudative tonsillitis. The typical presentation has been described, but in addition patients may complain of headaches and referred pain to the ear or neck. Malaise, dehydration and trismus are common features. Cultures from aspirates often show mixed aerobic and anaerobic organisms, the commonest being *Streptococcus pyogenes*.

The initial management involves:

- analgesia
- intravenous fluid administration for dehydration
- administration of broad-spectrum antibiotics
- consideration of intravenous steroids if severe or risk of airway compromise
- needle aspiration of abscess.

! Differential diagnoses

- Peritonsillitis
- Pharyngitis/parapharyngeal abscess
- Dental infection
- Infective mononucleosis
- Lymphoma
- Internal carotid artery aneurysm
- Other causes of para-pharyngeal swellings, e.g. salivary gland mass, infection, calculi

KEY POINT

- Although rare, patients with a quinsy can present with acute respiratory compromise necessitating prompt assessment by an ear, nose and throat and/or anaesthetic specialist.

CASE 83: EPISTAXIS

History

A 71-year-old woman attends the emergency department with a severe nose bleed. The bleeding started an hour before and is causing the patient a great deal of distress. She is not known to have any bleeding abnormalities. Previous medical history includes hypertension, angina and hypercholesterolaemia. She takes aspirin 75 mg od, bendrofluazide 2.5 mg od, isosorbide mononitrate 30 mg bd and simvastatin 40 mg nocte. She has no known allergies and she is an ex-smoker.

Examination

Her blood pressure is 172/103 mmHg and her pulse rate is 91/min. The oropharynx appears normal, with no evidence of blood draining in the posterior pharynx. Inspection of the nasal cavity using a speculum and light source suggests a bleeding point from the left nostril. There are no masses seen and there is no palpable cervical lymphadenopathy. The cardiovascular and respiratory examinations are normal.

INVESTIGATIONS

		Normal
Haemoglobin	12.3 g/L	11.5–16.0 g/dL
White cell count	8.0 × 10^9/L	4.0–11.0 × 10^9/L
Platelets	209 × 10^9/L	150–400 × 10^9/L
Coagulation profile: normal		

Questions

- How is epistaxis classified?
- What is Little's area?
- What is the aetiology?
- What is the basic management of epistaxis?

ANSWER 83

Epistaxis is defined as acute haemorrhage from the nasal cavity or nasopharynx. It is classified into anterior (anterior nasal cavity) or posterior (posterior nasal cavity and nasopharynx). Anterior bleeding is more common. It is commoner in the winter months when upper respiratory tract infections are more frequent.

Little's area refers to Kiesselbach's plexus, a network of blood vessels on the anterior portion of the nasal septum (feeding vessels from superior labial, greater palatine and anterior ethmoid arteries). This is the commonest point of bleeding in the anterior nasal cavity. Posterior bleeding tends to occur from branches of the sphenopalatine artery in the posterior nasal cavity or nasopharynx.

! Aetiology

- *Local*:
  - idiopathic
  - local trauma, e.g. nose picking/nasal bone fracture
  - iatrogenic, e.g. nasopharyngeal/ nasogastric intubation
  - infection/inflammation, e.g. upper respiratory tract infection/sinusitis/rhinitis
  - neoplasia
  - septal perforation/deviation
  - vascular anomalies, e.g. arterio-venous malformation, telangectasia
  - foreign body
  - irritants, e.g. chemicals, cigarette smoke, recreational drug use
- *Systemic*:
  - hypertension
  - bleeding disorders, e.g. haemophilia, platelet dysfunction, thromobocytopenia
  - leukaemia
  - liver disease, e.g. cirrhosis
  - medication, e.g. non-steroidal anti-inflammatory drugs, aspirin, heparin, warfarin

The basic management involves:

- an assessment of the patient's airway, breathing and circulation. Severe epistaxis may require endotracheal intubation. This is extremely rare
- manual compression of the nasal cavity (cartilaginous part of the nose) by asking the patient to grasp their nose and sustain pressure continuously for 10 min in an attempt to arrest the bleeding. Position the patient upright and ask him/her to lean forward over a bowl to try and avoid swallowing blood
- regular observations
- obtaining intravenous access and commencing intravenous fluids in patients with significant haemorrhage
- taking blood for a haemoglobin estimation, coagulation profile, and a crossmatch in cases of significant haemorrhage
- views can be improved by putting pledgets soaked with vasoconstrictor/local anaesthetic into the nose. This may help to identify the site of bleeding
- if a bleeding site is identified, a silver nitrate stick can be applied to the bleeding point to try to cauterize the bleeding after the administration of topical local anaesthetic
- if the above measures prove unsuccessful, the anterior part of the nose should be packed with nasal tampons. Both sides are packed, even in unilateral bleeding, as this provides better tamponade. An urgent ear, nose and throat (ENT) review should be requested if bleeding persists.

KEY POINTS

- Epistaxis can be life-threatening.
- If initial measures fail to control the bleeding, an ENT specialist should be sought.

CASE 84: STRIDOR

History

An 18-month-old baby girl is bought to the emergency department by her parents, as they are concerned about her noisy breathing. She has had a mild cough for the last 24 h and her temperature is elevated. She is up to date with her vaccinations and has had no developmental problems. There is no other relevant history.

Examination

Her oxygen saturation is 94 per cent on air. The baby is restless and has a hoarse cry. There is an audible stridor at rest. The baby has a low-grade fever with a mildly increased respiratory rate. There is no evidence of cyanosis. Auscultation of the chest is difficult but there is an audible inspiratory noise.

Questions

- What is the differential diagnosis?
- How do you define stridor?
- What are the causes of stridor?

ANSWER 84

In this case the two most likely diagnoses are croup (acute laryngo-tracheo-bronchitis) or acute epiglottitis. Laryngo-tracheo-bronchitis presents in childhood and is usually preceded by an upper respiratory tract infection. The child develops malaise, a high temperature and stridor. The stridor is the result of subglottic oedema which soon spreads to the trachea and bronchi. It is usually caused by a viral infection (parainfluenza). Mild cases of croup often respond to oral steroids. Severe cases may require ventilatory support as well as nebulized adrenaline and inhaled or intravenous steroids.

Acute epiglottitis is an absolute emergency and is usually caused by *Haemophilus influenzae*. There is significant swelling and any attempt to examine the throat may result in airway obstruction. It is rare in children these days because they receive the Haemophilus influenzae type B (HiB) vaccination aspart of their routine immunization programme. In adults it tends to cause a supraglottitis. It has a rapid progression and can lead to total airway obstruction. The patient must be sat upright and an airway secured with an endotracheal tube, by an anaesthetic specialist.

Stridor is defined as a high-pitched noise caused by turbulent airflow in the larynx or trachea as the result of narrowing of the airway.

! Aetiology of stridor

- *Neonate:*
  - laryngomalacia/tracheomalacia
  - vocal cord lesion/palsy, e.g. neurological, birth/surgical trauma
  - laryngotracheal stenosis, e.g. congenital
  - airway haemangioma
- *Child*:
  - croup
  - acute epiglottitis
  - airway haemangioma
  - foreign body
  - trauma
  - airway compression, e.g. thyroid disease
- *Adult*:
  - vocal cord palsy secondary to thyroid or chest surgery
  - acute epiglottitis/supraglottitis
  - laryngeal carcinoma
  - laryngotracheal stenosis, e.g. secondary to endotracheal intubation or heat inhalation
  - inhalation of a foreign body
  - trauma to the anterior neck
  - airway compression by thyroid disease

KEY POINTS

- Stridor is an ominous sign and needs to be taken seriously.
- Treatment is urgent and the patient should be managed in a suitable area, e.g. theatre, resuscitation bay.
- Call for ear, nose and throat and anaesthetic help early.

CASE 85: FACIAL WEAKNESS

History

A 42-year-old man attends the emergency department complaining of weakness down one side of his face. Over the last 2 days, he has noticed an altered taste sensation and pain in and around the ear on the same side. There is no history of trauma. He has not noticed any discharge from the ear and there is no limb weakness. He is a known asthmatic and he suffers with depression. He has recently given up smoking and has spent several weeks in India on holiday with his wife. He is currently using salbutamol and becotide inhalers and takes paroxetine 20 mg od. He has no known allergies.

Examination

Cardiovascular, respiratory and abdominal examinations are normal. His gait and balance are normal. Neurology of the upper and lower limbs is unremarkable. Examining the face you notice some asymmetry, which is more obvious when you ask the patient to smile. When you ask him to show his teeth, the right side of the face droops. On raising his eyebrows, there is a loss of the forehead facial wrinkles on the right and he has difficulty in closing his right eye. The rest of the cranial nerves appear intact and examination of the ear is normal. There is no evidence of trauma and the salivary glands feel normal.

Questions

- Which nerve has been affected?
- Does this represent an upper or lower motor neurone lesion?
- What is the differential diagnosis?
- What is the treatment in this case?

ANSWER 85

The patient has a lower motor neurone right-sided facial nerve palsy. The unilateral paresis of the facial muscles makes it difficult for the patient to close the eye on that side and the mouth droops on smiling. The forehead wrinkles are also lost when the patient raises the eyebrows and there is loss of the nasolabial fold.

The facial paresis would have spared the upper facial muscles if the patient had an upper motor neurone lesion (UMN), i.e. a lesion proximal to the facial nucleus located in the pons. The upper facial muscles receive a bilateral cortical innervation, so their function is maintained by the intact contralateral nerve supply in an UMN lesion.

! Differential diagnoses

- *Upper motor neurone lesion*:
  - cerebrovascular accident
  - cerebral tumour
  - multiple sclerosis
  - motor neurone disease
- *Lower motor neurone lesion*:
  - idiopathic, i.e. Bell's palsy
  - Ramsay Hunt syndrome, i.e. Herpes zoster infection of the facial nerve
  - acute otitis media
  - cholesteatoma
  - trauma, e.g. fracture of the temporal bone, surgery
  - parotid mass, e.g. carcinoma
  - cerebello-pontine angle tumour, e.g. acoustic neuroma

Bell's palsy is diagnosed when other lower motor neurone pathologies have been excluded. It is the most likely diagnosis in this case. The aetiology is thought to be viral and secondary to inflammation within the facial nerve.

Initial treatment is:

- steroids, e.g. prednisolone within 48 h of symptoms
- consider antiviral therapy, e.g. aciclovir
- eye protection as the patient will not be able to blink.

KEY POINT

- The forehead is spared in upper motor neurone lesions.

NEUROSURGERY

CASE 86: THUNDERCLAP HEADACHE

History

A 56-year-old woman is brought to the emergency department by her partner. She had initially complained of a severe headache before collapsing unconscious on the floor at home. She has no significant past medical history but smokes 30 cigarettes a day. She has now regained consciousness and is complaining of neck stiffness. Her initial assessment is carried out using the system shown below.

Examination

Eye opening		**Best motor response**		**Best verbal response**	
1 None	☐	1 None	☐	1 None	☐
2 To pain	☐	2 Extension to pain	☐	2 Incomprehensible sounds	☐
3 To speech	☒	3 Flexion to pain	☐	3 Inappropriate words	☐
4 Spontaneous	☐	4 Withdraws from pain	☐	4 Confused	☒
		5 Localizes to pain	☐	5 Orientated	☐
		6 Obeys commands	☒		
				Score 13/15	

Questions

- What system has been used to assess the patient?
- What is the likely diagnosis?
- What are the possible underlying causes?

ANSWER 86

The Glasgow Coma Score (GCS) is composed of three parameters: verbal commands, eye opening and motor responses. The patient is assessed on their 'best' response. The scores are summed to give an overall value from 3 (being the worst) to 15 (being the best). In this case the GCS is 13. While the score is useful in absolute terms, such as defining coma (GCS $\leq$8), the main value of the GCS is being able to monitor the ongoing neurological status of a patient by repeated assessment every 15 min. A fall in the score of 2 or more should prompt an urgent review of the patient, as this indicates a potentially significant deterioration in their condition.

The most likely diagnosis in this case is of a subarachnoid haemorrhage. The classical symptoms are of a severe 'thunderclap' headache affecting the back of the head that reaches maximal intensity within a few seconds.

! Causes of bleeding into the subarachnoid space

- 85 per cent: saccular aneurysms in the cerebral vasculature – 'berry' aneurysms
- 15 per cent: non-aneursymal subarachnoid haemorrhage:
  - arterial dissection
  - arteriovenous malformation
  - tumour
  - cocaine abuse
  - trauma
  - septic aneurysm

The initial management involves stabilizing the patient and arranging the following:

- *blood tests*: full blood count, renal function, coagulation screen and group and save
- *computerized tomography (CT) of the brain*: to look for evidence of subarachnoid blood and hydrocephalus
- *lumbar puncture*: if the CT scan does not show any pathology, then cerebral spinal fluid should be sent for spectrophotometric analysis to look for the presence of oxyhaemoglobin and bilirubin.

Differential diagnoses include transient ischaemic attacks, migraine or epilepsy. Patients confirmed to have a subarachnoid haemorrhage should be referred to a neurosurgical unit for further assessment (cerebral angiography) and treatment (embolization).

KEY POINTS

- The Glasgow Coma Score ranges from 3 to 15.
- A fall of 2 points or more should prompt immediate reassessment.

CASE 87: CONFUSION AFTER A FALL

History

You are asked to review a 78-year-old man on the observation ward. He was admitted the previous evening with confusion. Earlier in the evening a friend visited and reported that he had fallen over 3 weeks ago and had become increasingly confused and clumsy.

He takes a calcium antagonist for essential hypertension and aspirin since a previous heart attack. He lives alone and is independent and self-caring. He is a non-smoker, but there had been concerns over his increasing alcohol intake following the death of his wife 5 years ago.

Examination

He has a normal temperature with a pulse rate of 78/min and a blood pressure of 136/86 mmHg. The cardiorespiratory and abdominal systems appear normal. He is confused in time, place and person. His pupils are symmetrical and reactive. The rest of his cranial nerve and peripheral neurological examinations are normal.

INVESTIGATIONS

See Fig. 87.1.

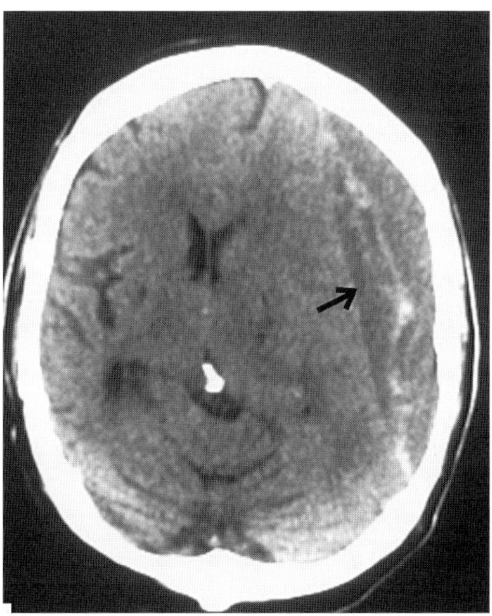

Figure 87.1 Imaging of the head. (Reproduced with kind permission from Liebenberg W. A. et al 2006. *Neurosurgery Explained*. Vesuvius Books Ltd.)

Questions

- What investigation is shown and what is the diagnosis?
- Which factors in the history make you suspicious of this diagnosis?

ANSWER 87

This man has a chronic subdural haematoma (CSDH) shown on a computerized tomography (CT) scan (arrow in Fig. 87.1). This condition is twice as common in men as women. Risk factors include chronic alcoholism, epilepsy, anticoagulant therapy (including aspirin) and thrombocytopenia.

CSDH is commonly associated with cerebral atrophy. It is thought that cortical bridging veins are under greater tension as the brain gradually shrinks away from the skull. He has had a head injury in the preceding weeks. Minor trauma can cause one of the cortical veins to tear. Slow bleeding from the low-pressure venous system often allows a large haematoma to form before clinical signs become evident.

Initial misdiagnosis is, unfortunately, quite common. Before the advent of CT scanning, CSDH was known as the 'great imitator' as it was often mistaken for dementia, transient ischaemic attacks or strokes.

The CT findings for subdural haematomas change with time. In the first week, the blood is hyperdense compared to brain tissue. In the second and third weeks, the haematoma appears isodense compared to brain tissue, and after the third week, the blood appears hypodense compared to brain tissue.

The term chronic is applied to subdural haematomas that are older than 21 days. When there is no clear history of a head injury (25–50 per cent of patients), the diagnosis can be made radiologically according to the CT appearances of the blood.

Once the diagnosis is made, the liquefied blood can be drained via one or two Burr holes. Even for patients with significant comorbidities, operative intervention is not contraindicated as this procedure can be performed under local anaesthetic. Eighty per cent of patients will return to their previous level of function.

KEY POINTS

- The clinical signs of a chronic subdural haematoma can be subtle.
- A chronic subdural haematoma should be suspected in confused patients with a history of a fall.

CASE 88: HEAD TRAUMA

History

A 17-year-old boy is brought to the emergency department by ambulance. He had been playing hockey and was struck on the head by a hockey ball approximately half an hour before admission. He lost consciousness briefly, but was able to walk from the scene. He is mildly confused, complaining of a severe headache, and has vomited four times.

Examination

He has a pulse rate of 63/min and a blood pressure of 170/110 mmHg. During the course of the examination he becomes drowsy and his Glasgow Coma Score (GCS) drops to 3/15. He has a 'boggy swelling' over the right temple. His right pupil is dilated.

INVESTIGATIONS

A computerized tomography (CT) scan of the head is shown in Fig. 88.1.

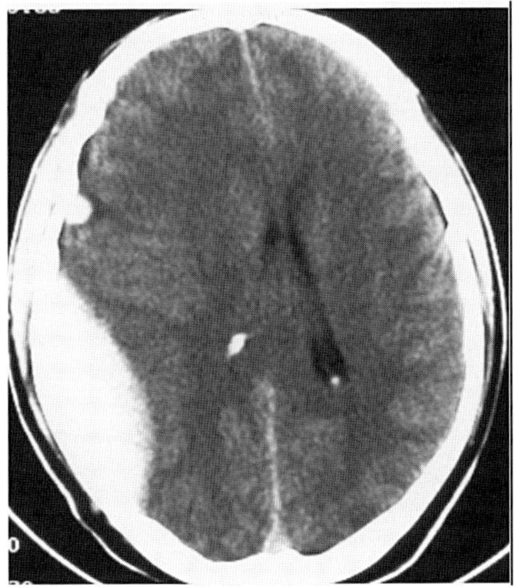

Figure 88.1 Computerized tomography scan of the head. (Reproduced with kind permission from Liebenberg W. A. et al 2006. *Neurosurgery Explained*. Vesuvius Books Ltd.)

Questions

- What is the diagnosis?
- What is the explanation for his vital signs?
- How should this patient be managed?

ANSWER 88

This young man has sustained an extradural bleed. A direct blow to the temporo-parietal area is the commonest cause of an extradural haematoma. The bleed is normally arterial in origin. In 85 per cent of cases there is an associated skull fracture that causes damage to the middle meningeal artery. Only 20 per cent of patients have the classic presentation of a lucid interval between the initial trauma and subsequent neurological deterioration.

The Cushing response refers to the presence of hypertension with an associated bradycardia resulting from raised intracranial pressure. The skull can be thought of as a closed box with no room for expansion, so when there is an arterial bleed, the pressure inside the 'box' increases rapidly. The CT scan demonstrates the hyperdense (white) appearance of an acute haematoma (arrow in Fig. 88.2). The location of the haematoma is in the 'potential' space between the skull and dural membrane. Expansion of the blood produces the smooth-margined convex mass seen on the image compressing the brain tissue.

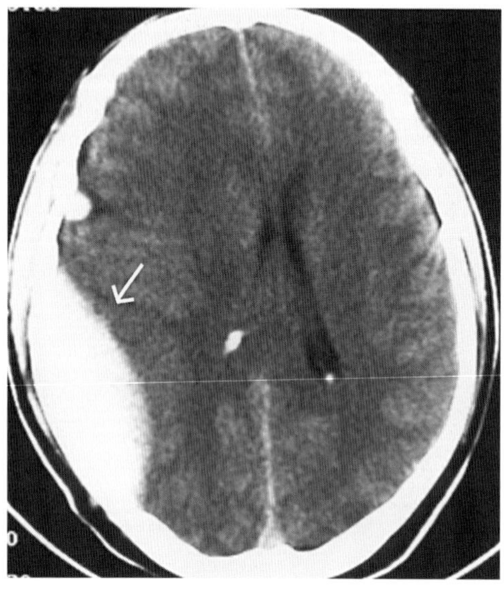

Figure 88.2 Computerized tomography showing an extradural haematoma (arrow). (Reproduced with kind permission from Liebenberg W. A. et al 2006. *Neurosurgery Explained*. Vesuvius Books Ltd.)

The pressure created has shifted the midline and compressed the ventricular system. Further increases in pressure can only be accommodated by downward herniation of the brainstem through the foramen magnum. The resulting brainstem ischaemia is thought to lead to the Cushing response.

This situation represents a neurosurgical emergency. Without urgent decompression the patient will die. Unlike the chronic subdural, which can be treated with Burr hole drainage, the more dense acute arterial haematoma requires a craniotomy in order to evacuate it. The GCS of 3/15 would indicate that this patient is unlikely to be able to maintain his own airway and will almost certainly require intubation and ventilation prior to CT scanning.

KEY POINTS

- Only 20 per cent of patients have the classical lucid interval.
- Extradural haematomas are most commonly caused by damage to the middle meningeal artery.

CASE 89: LOWER BACK PAIN

History

A 40-year-old man presents to his general practitioner with lower back pain and pain radiating down his right leg. The pain started as he was lifting a wardrobe in the bedroom. Since then he has also noticed that his foot feels 'strange', and he catches it every time he walks up stairs. On direct questioning he says he feels slightly bloated and hasn't passed urine since the morning. He is normally fit and healthy. He takes no regular medication. He smokes 5 cigars a day and drinks 30 units of alcohol a week. He is married and works as a structural engineer.

Examination

His vital signs are normal. Abdominal examination reveals a palpable mass in the suprapubic region. Examination of the lumbar spine is normal. The power in his legs is reduced, with weakness of ankle dorsiflexion and the extensor hallucis longus. He has reduced pinprick sensation over the lateral aspect of his right foot. The sensation around his perineum is abnormal. He has an absent ankle reflex on the right. A digital rectal examination reveals reduced anal tone. His pedal pulses are palpable.

Questions

- What is the likely diagnosis?
- What are the initial stages in this man's management?
- What investigation should be arranged?

ANSWER 89

This man has cauda equina syndrome.

The spinal cord tapers and ends at the level between the first and second lumbar vertebrae in the average adult. The most distal part of the spinal cord is called the conus medullaris, and its tapering end continues as the filum terminale. Distal to the end of the spinal cord are the nerve roots, which have the appearance of a horse's tail, hence the latin term 'cauda equina'.

Cauda equina syndrome occurs when there is compression of the nerve roots at this level. There are a number of causes including traumatic injury, spinal stenosis, spinal neoplasm, schwannomas, ependymomas, inflammatory conditions, and infection. However, as in this case, the likely cause is intervertebral disc herniation, which is the responsible for up to 15 per cent of cases. Over 90 per cent of disc herniations occur at the L4–L5 or L5–S1 levels.

The important features in this case are the presence of urogenital signs and symptoms. The palpable suprapubic mass is his bladder, as he has developed urinary retention. The abnormal sensation around his perineum, which is typically described as 'saddle anaesthesia', is pathognomonic. A digital rectal examination is useful in determining anal tone and is also used to determine the severity of the neurological compromise.

It should be possible to accurately determine the level of neurological compromise by detailed neurological examination (Table 89.1). An urgent magnetic resonance imaging (MRI) scan of the lumbar spine is performed to give detailed information regarding the exact location and nature of the pathology. The patient should be referred urgently to a spinal centre once the diagnosis has been confirmed.

Table 89.1 Summary of the clinical findings in lower-limb neurological disease

Nerve root	Sensory deficit	Motor deficit	Reduced reflexes
L2	Antero-lateral thigh	Hip flexion	
L3	Medial thigh and knee	Quadriceps weakness and knee extension	Knee
L4	Medial calf and malleolus	Knee extension	Knee
L5	Dorsum of foot and lateral calf	Extensor hallucis longus	Ankle
S1–S2	Lateral foot	Plantar flexion of foot	Ankle
S3–S4	Saddle region	Sphincters	Anal

KEY POINTS

- 90 per cent of disc herniations occur at the L4–L5/L5–S1 levels.
- An urgent MRI scan of the spine should be performed in any patient with back pain and urogenital signs or symptoms.

ANAESTHESIA

CASE 90: DAY CASE SURGERY

HISTORY

A 56-year-old man has been referred to the surgical outpatient department with a right-sided inguinal hernia. He has requested a day surgical procedure. The patient has type 2 diabetes and hypertension. He has no history of a myocardial infarction or angina. He lives in a house with 10 stairs, which he can climb easily without shortness of breath. He takes metformin 500 mg tds for his diabetes and atenolol 50 mg daily for his hypertension. He is a non-smoker and drinks fewer than 12 units of alcohol per week. He lives with his wife who is fit and independent.

Examination

His blood pressure is 130/80 mmHg and the pulse rate is 88/min. His body mass index (BMI) is 28 and a random blood sugar is 6 mmol/L. The chest is clear and heart sounds are normal. Abdominal examination reveals an easily reducible non-tender right inguinal hernia.

Questions

- Which factors are important in patients being considered for day surgery?
- What is the patient's ASA (American Society of Anaesthesiologists) status?
- Why are the patient's social circumstances important?
- What would you advise about the metformin prior to surgery?

ANSWER 90

The criteria for day-surgery selection are based on published guidelines and recommendations, which vary between hospital trusts. The surgical procedure should have an estimated operation time of less than 1 h with minimal expected blood loss. Operations that lead to severe postoperative pain or nausea are not suitable as day cases. Operations that lead to a loss of independence or toilet function are also unsuitable. The risk of complications should be minimized with the aim to prevent an inpatient stay. To determine a patient's fitness for surgery, the anaesthetists grade physical status using the American Society of Anaesthesiologists (ASA) classification:

- *Class 1*: patients with no organic, physiological, biochemical or psychiatric disturbance
- *Class 2*: patients with mild systemic disease but no functional limitations, e.g. controlled diabetes or hypertension
- *Class 3*: patients with moderate systemic disease and functional limitations
- *Class 4*: severe systemic disease which is a constant threat to life
- *Class 5*: moribund patient, not expected to survive 24 h.

Patients should ideally be ASA 1 or 2, but some units will accept 3, depending on the disease. This particular patient has an ASA of 2, as he has well-controlled systemic disease with no functional limitations. There is no absolute restriction on age, as the selection is mainly based on physical status. A patient should be able to climb a flight of stairs and should ideally have a BMI <35. Patients with uncontrolled hypertension, epilepsy, cardiac failure or severe gastric reflux are usually considered unsuitable.

Social criteria must also be met before patients can attend day surgery:

- the patient should be accompanied for the first 24–48 h after surgery
- an escort should be available to take the patient home
- the patient or carer must have access to a private telephone
- the travel time to home must not exceed 1.5 h.

Metformin should be stopped for up to 48 h prior to surgery. Lactic acidosis is a rare, serious metabolic complication that can occur from metformin accumulation, especially in patients with renal failure.

KEY POINTS

- The ASA system is used to grade a patient's fitness for surgery.
- Patients should be formally assessed for their suitability for day surgery.

CASE 91: ANTICOAGULATION

History

A 64-year-old woman attending the surgical pre-admission clinic, is due to be admitted in 2 weeks' time for an incisional hernia repair. She is known to have atrial fibrillation and is on warfarin. She has also had a recent exacerbation of her chronic obstructive airways disease for which the general practitioner has prescribed antibiotics and a one-week course of prednisolone (30 mg od). The treatment is due to be completed in a couple of days, and the anaesthetist has already seen her to organize further respiratory investigations.

Examination

She is a thin woman with a previous midline laparotomy scar. Her chest is clear and the heart sounds are normal. Examination of the abdomen confirms a large midline defect in the abdominal wall. The hernia is easily reducible and non-tender.

Questions

- How should the anticoagulation be managed prior to surgery?
- Is the recent course of steroids relevant?

ANSWER 91

It is important to determine the patient's risk of thromboembolic disease before discontinuing anticoagulation. Patients with a low risk of thrombosis should have their warfarin discontinued 4–5 days before surgery. Warfarin should be restarted at the preoperative dose at a safe interval after the procedure, depending on the operation. Patients with prosthetic valves, atrial fibrillation with mitral valve disease and patients with a history of thromboembolism are considered to be at high risk of further thrombosis. These patients should be admitted for heparin treatment prior to surgery. Heparin should be discontinued immediately prior to surgery and restarted postoperatively. The heparin should be continued until the warfarin has been restarted and reached its therapeutic level.

This patient has atrial fibrillation, with no other risk factors, so is considered to be low risk for thrombosis. It is also important to ask if a patient is on any other medication that may affect coagulation. The following agents should be stopped at the given time prior to surgery:

- *clopidogrel*: 7 days
- *ibuprofen*: 2 days
- *aspirin*: 7 to10 days
- *cilostazol*: 5 days.

In a normal individual there is a daily secretion of cortisol, which increases in response to illness or surgery. Patients on regular steroids have a suppressed hypothalamo-pituitary-adrenal axis, which leads to an impaired stress response. This can lead to hypotension and cardiovascular compromise after major surgery. The following patients should be considered for steroid replacement when undergoing a surgical procedure:

- patients on long-term corticosteroids at a dose of more than 10 mg prednisolone daily (or equivalent)
- patients who have received corticosteroids at a dose of more than 10 mg daily, in the last three months (the patient in this question will, therefore, require steroid-replacement therapy)
- patients taking high-dose inhalation corticosteroids (e.g. beclometasone 1.5 mg a day).

Patients having a minor procedure, such as an inguinal hernia repair, require a bolus of hydrocortisone at induction. Patients admitted for a moderate procedure, such as laparoscopic cholecystectomy, require additional 8-hourly doses of hydrocortisone for 24–48 h postoperatively. Patients for a major procedure require intravenous steroids for at least 2 days postoperatively.

KEY POINTS

- Anticoagulation should be stopped prior to surgery.
- Patients on steroids may require steroid replacement peri- and postoperatively.

CASE 92: FITNESS FOR SURGERY – CARDIAC DISEASE

History

At the preoperative assessment clinic, you have been asked to clerk a 76-year-old man for a total hip replacement. He has been placed on the waiting list by the consultant 3 months previously. He currently walks with two sticks and is woken at night with pain in his right hip. Since his initial consultation, the patient has had intermittent episodes of chest tightness and dizziness brought on by exertion. The symptoms subside with rest and have been associated with pain in the left arm. He was seen in the emergency department the previous week after an episode of collapse and was told he may have suffered a heart attack. He is now waiting to see his general practitioner (GP) for further investigation.

He has no previous history of heart disease and was, up until recently, able to climb the 12 steps to his flat without shortness of breath. He is currently taking aspirin, which was started by the emergency department doctor after his collapse. He does not smoke and has the occasional social drink.

Examination

The patient's blood pressure is 186/106 mmHg and the pulse rate is 84/min. On auscultation, the chest is clear, but there is a systolic murmur over the right sternal edge which radiates into the neck. Examination of the right hip demonstrates limited internal rotation, compared to the left side.

INVESTIGATIONS

		Normal
Haemoglobin	12.0 g/dL	11.5–16.0 g/dL
Mean cell volume	82 fL	76–96 fL
White cell count	10.2×10^9/L	$4.0–11.0 \times 10^9$/L
Platelets	250×10^9/L	$150–400 \times 10^9$/L
Sodium	138 mmol/L	135–145 mmol/L
Potassium	3.6 mmol/L	3.5–5.0 mmol/L
Urea	5.2 mmol/L	2.5–6.7 mmmol/L
Creatinine	76 μmol/L	44–80 μmol/L

Questions

- What concerns do you have about this patient's fitness for surgery?
- Which investigations should be ordered before proceeding with surgery?
- Do any other specialists need to be consulted about this patient's care prior to surgery?

ANSWER 92

The patient has clinical evidence of serious cardiac disease and is an extremely high risk for an elective surgical procedure. The patient's history and examination have highlighted a number of important risk factors:

- *hypertension*: he is hypertensive, which is associated with an increased incidence of ischemia, left ventricular dysfunction, arrhythmia and stroke during the perioperative period. Patients should ideally have a systolic blood pressure of less than 140 mmHg and a diastolic blood pressure of less than 90 mmHg before proceeding with surgery. This patient should be referred back to his GP or to a specialist for antihypertensive medication
- *ischemic heart disease*: it is important to establish whether this patient did have a heart attack the previous week. An electrocardiogram or a troponin T, taken 12 h after the collapse, may provide evidence of a myocardial infarct. Patients having an operation within 3 months of a myocardial infarction carry a 30 per cent risk of reinfarction or cardiac death. This drops to 5 per cent after 6 months. The patient also appears to be suffering from angina, which needs further investigation by a cardiologist prior to surgery. Patients with acute coronary syndrome carry a significant risk of perioperative myocardial infarction and may benefit from a revascularization procedure
- *aortic stenosis*: the systolic murmur radiating to the carotid may be due to aortic stenosis. Aortic stenosis leads to overload of the left ventricle, resulting in ventricular hypertrophy and ultimately dilatation and failure. The severity of the valvular disease can be assessed by echocardiography. The patient may require valve replacement prior to hip replacement if there is evidence of a tight stenosis of the aortic valve. If left undiagnosed, it is associated with a 10-fold increase of perioperative death. This patient's high blood pressure makes a significant stenosis unlikely.

KEY POINT

- Patients having an operation within 3 months of a myocardial infarction carry a 30 per cent risk of reinfarction.

CASE 93: FITNESS FOR SURGERY – RESPIRATORY ASSESSMENT

History

You are the doctor in the surgical pre-assessment clinic. Your first patient is a 66-year-old man who is being admitted for an elective abdomino-perineal resection for rectal carcinoma. He suffers with chronic obstructive pulmonary disease (COPD) and is a smoker of 15 cigarettes a day. Apart from mild hypertension there is no evidence of cardiac disease. He uses inhalers daily and takes oral theophyhlline and amlodopine. His exercise tolerance is 30 yards and he has had two previous admissions to hospital with breathing problems. He has never required admission to an intensive-care unit. He does not require home oxygen at present. His father died of lung cancer. He currently lives alone.

Examination

His blood pressure is 146/92 mmHg, pulse rate 88/min and oxygen saturations are 93 per cent on air. The heart sounds are normal. On auscultation of the chest there is moderate air entry with some scattered wheeze. The rest of the examination is unremarkable.

Questions

- What tests would you consider organizing in addition to routine bloods and an electrocardiogram?
- What are the potential problems that patients with significant COPD face in the postoperative period?
- What advice would you give him regarding his smoking habit prior to his surgery?

ANSWER 93

This patient will need an up-to-date chest X-ray, a baseline arterial blood gas and some basic respiratory function tests, such as spirometry. Spirometry is a timed measurement of dynamic lung volumes during forced expiration, used to quantify lung capacity and determine how quickly the lungs can be emptied. The measurements usually taken are the forced vital capacity, forced expiratory volume in one second and the ratio of these two volumes (FEV_1/FVC). A ratio of <70 per cent indicates an obstructive ventilatory defect, such as COPD. Patients with restrictive airways disease, such as interstitial lung disease or kyphoscoliosis, have smaller volumes and tend to have a ratio of >80 per cent.

Patients with COPD have difficulty clearing secretions from the lungs during the postoperative period. They also have a higher risk of basal atelectasis and are more prone to chest infections. These factors in combination with postoperative pain (especially in thoracic or abdominal major surgery) make them prone to respiratory complications. Consultation with a chest physiotherapist both prior to surgery, to teach breathing exercises, and in the postoperative period in order to optimize respiratory function is essential. Adequate analgesia is essential postoperatively and often requires the use of an epidural. Patients should also be taught how to hold their incisions to prevent pain when taking deep breaths or coughing.

Summary of complications more common in those with preoperative respiratory disease

- Atelectasis
- Bronchospasm
- Chest infection
- Hypoxia
- Pulmonary embolism
- Respiratory failure

Every effort must be made to persuade patients who smoke to give up prior to surgery. Those with lung disease will benefit if this is done at least 6 weeks before an operation. There is a reduction in mucus hypersecretion, small-airway narrowing and an improvement in tracheo-bronchial clearance of secretions. Patients with cardiac disease should also be encouraged to stop smoking prior to surgery. The increased carbon monoxide levels and the effects of nicotine (increased heart rate and systemic blood pressure) lead to an increase in cardiac stress during surgery. This can be significantly improved if smoking is stopped 24 h prior to surgery, due to the short half-lives of nicotine and carbon monoxide.

KEY POINTS

- Patients with COPD are more prone to basal atelectasis and chest infections.
- Patients should be encouraged to give up smoking at least 6 weeks prior to surgery.

CASE 94: FITNESS FOR SURGERY – PATIENTS WITH DIABETES

History

You are the surgical doctor in the pre-assessment clinic and you are asked to review a 56-year-old man who is due to have a transurethral resection of a bladder tumour (TURBT). He has non-insulin-dependent diabetes and had a myocardial infarction 7 years ago. His current medications include metformin 500 mg bd, gliclazide 80 mg od, aspirin 75 mg od, lisinopril 20 mg od and gaviscon prn. He has no known allergies. He gave up smoking after his myocardial infarction.

Examination

Observations are normal. The patient appears comfortable. Heart sounds are normal and the chest is clear. The abdomen is soft, non-tender and the genitalia are normal.

Questions

- Which investigations would be appropriate prior to his surgery?
- What types of complications commonly affect patients with diabetes?
- Where should the patient be placed on the operating list?
- What regimen would you recommend for keeping good glycaemic control in the peri- and postoperative period?

ANSWER 94

The patient should have a full blood count, urea and electrolytes and a haemoglobin A_{1c} as an indicator of previous glycaemic control. When assessing patients with diabetes in pre-assessment, a full cardiovascular, respiratory, abdominal and neurological examination should be performed. The lower limbs should be examined for peripheral neuropathy and ulceration. The peripheral pulses should also be palpated for evidence of peripheral vascular disease. Fundoscopy should be carried out to assess the retina, and a blood pressure measurement should be recorded in both the lying and standing positions to assess for autonomic neuropathy. An electrocardiogram should be done to screen for cardiac disease.

Patients with diabetes have an increased risk of postoperative complications because of the presence of micro- and macrovascular disease:

- *atherosclerosis*: ischaemic heart disease/peripheral vascular disease/cerebrovascular disease
- *nephropathy*: renal insufficiency
- *retinopathy*: limited visual acuity
- *autonomic neuropathy*: gastroparesis, decreased bladder tone
- *peripheral neuropathy*: lower-extremity ulceration, infection, gangrene
- *poor wound healing*
- *increased risk of infection.*

Tight glycaemic control (6–10 mmol/L) and the prevention of hypoglycaemia are critical in preventing peri- and postoperative complications. The patient with diabetes should be placed first on the operating list to avoid prolonged fasting. For patients with insulin-dependent diabetes, a 'sliding scale' regimen of insulin is given at a particular rate according to the blood glucose. Patients with diet-controlled diabetes who are undergoing minor surgery need no specific treatment. Those undergoing minor surgery whose diabetes is controlled with oral hypoglycaemic agents should omit their medication prior to surgery to prevent hypoglycaemia or lactic acidosis. They should recommence once they are eating and drinking properly after their surgery. Those that are having major surgery but are expected to be able to eat and drink relatively soon postoperatively can have a trial of omitting their medication on the morning of surgery and close blood glucose monitoring. If the blood glucose is greater than 12 mmol/L prior to surgery, or where feeding is not likely to start soon after surgery, a 'sliding scale' insulin regimen should be instigated. Some patients will be taking chlorpropramide, a long-acting sulphonylurea for diabetic control. This should be stopped 48 h prior to surgery to prevent hypoglycaemia in the peri- and postoperative period.

KEY POINTS

- Insulin-dependent patients should be placed on a sliding scale prior to fasting.
- Oral hypoglycaemic agents should be stopped prior to surgery.

POSTOPERATIVE COMPLICATIONS

CASE 95: NUTRITION

History

On the ward round with your consultant, you see a patient on intensive care. The patient had an emergency laparotomy for faecal peritonitis 5 days previously. He underwent a Hartmann's procedure for a perforated sigmoid diverticulitis. He is currently being ventilated and has developed a hospital-acquired pneumonia. He is likely to require ventilation on intensive care for a number of days and the staff are concerned because he has not received any nutrition since his operation.

Questions

- What are the two main methods of providing nutrition that you may consider?
- What are the routes of administration for each type?
- What are the advantages and disadvantages of each type?
- What is a Hartmann's procedure?
- Which method of feeding would be most appropriate in this patient?

ANSWER 95

Malnutrition leads to delayed wound healing, reduced ventilatory capacity, reduced immunity and an increased risk of infection. The nutritional status of a patient should be assessed daily.

The two main methods of feeding are either by the enteral route or the parenteral route.

Enteral feeding is via the gastrointestinal tract. It is less expensive and is associated with fewer complications than feeding by the parenteral route. Enteral feeding stimulates the bowel and encourages the production of mucosal factors which maintain the normal physiological barrier to bacterial translocation. Patients who can take food orally can have their diet supplemented with nutritional drinks. If patients are not able to feed orally, then nasoenteral tube feeding should be considered. Nasogastric feeding is the mostly commonly used route. Tube tips can be placed in the duodenum or jejunum if there is pathology in the proximal part of the gastrointestinal tract. In the longer term, enteral feeding can be via a feeding gastrostomy or jejunostomy. These can be placed either endoscopically, radiologically or at the time of surgery. Disadvantages are that feeding tubes can become blocked or dislodged, leading to peritonitis.

The parenteral route should only be used if there is an inability to ingest, digest, absorb or propulse nutrients through the gastrointestinal tract. It can be administered by either a peripheral or central line. Peripheral parenteral nutrition can cause thrombophlebitis due to the hyperosmotic nature of the feed. Central parenteral nutrition needs to be delivered via a large central line – in the subclavian or jugular vein. Insertion of a central line carries a significant risk of complications, e.g. pneumothorax, haematoma, nerve injury and thrombosis. Sepsis is the most frequent and serious complication of centrally administered parenteral nutrition. The other serious complication relates to metabolic derangement, which occurs in up to 5 per cent of patients on parenteral nutrition.

A Hartmann's procedure is a safe method of removing a diseased section of large bowel. After resection, the distal part of the bowel is closed and left *in situ*, and the proximal end is brought to the skin as an end colostomy. There is no anastamosis, which allows enteral nutrition to be started early.

KEY POINTS

- Enteral feeding is preferred to parenteral feeding.
- A patient's nutritional status should be assessed on a daily basis.

CASE 96: POSTOPERATIVE PYREXIA

History

As the doctor on call, you have been asked to assess an 86-year-old patient on the ward who is 1 day post perforated peptic ulcer repair. The nurse is concerned as he has spiked a temperature. The operations note reports that there was minimal peritoneal soiling at the time of the operation. He has a morphine infusion, but his pain is poorly controlled. A urinary catheter remains from his operation and the urine output is adequate. Prior to his surgery he was fit, but he was a heavy smoker.

Examination

His blood pressure is 130/90 mmHg, pulse rate 110/min, respiratory rate 30/min and temperature 38°C. His saturations have remained at 99 per cent on 24 per cent oxygen. On examination of his chest you can hear coarse basal crepitations bilaterally and the lung bases are dull on percussion. Abdominal examination reveals tenderness around the incision site and the urinalysis is clear. Blood tests and a portable chest X-ray (Fig. 96.1) are ordered and shown below.

INVESTIGATIONS

		Normal
Haemoglobin	10.5 g/dL	11.5–16.0 g/dL
Mean cell volume	80 fL	76–96 fL
White cell count	12.2×10^9/L	$4.0–11.0 \times 10^9$/L
Platelets	250×10^9/L	$150–400 \times 10^9$/L
Sodium	138 mmol/L	135–145 mmol/L
Potassium	3.6 mmol/L	3.5–5.0 mmol/L
Urea	5 mmol/L	2.5–6.7 mmmol/L
Creatinine	52 μmol/L	44–80 μmol/L

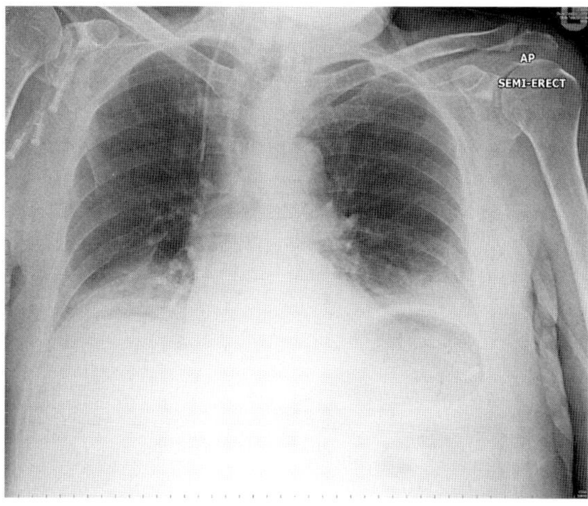

Figure 96.1 Plain X-ray of the chest.

Questions

- What is the likely cause of the pyrexia in this patient?
- What are the risk factors?
- How should the patient be managed?

ANSWER 96

The chest X-ray shows a reduction in lung volume bilaterally, and basal consolidation. The patient has basal atelectasis as a consequence of pulmonary collapse. The patient's inability to cough leads to the failure of clearance of bronchial secretions from the lungs. Consequently, there is occlusion and collapse of the lung segments. The collapsed lung is at risk of secondary infection by inhaled organisms, leading to a pneumonia.

Atelectasis is more common in patients with pre-existing lung disease, obese patients and heavy smokers. Patients who have undergone thoracic or upper-abdominal surgery find chest expansion limited by pain, making them more prone to basal lung collapse. The patient in this case has a number of risk factors for developing basal atelectasis. He is a heavy smoker and has an upper midline incision with poor postoperative pain control.

Patients with basal atelectasis usually develop a pyrexia at about 48 h, with an accompanying tachycardia and tachypnoea. Examination reveals bronchial breathing, and reduced air entry bibasally with dullness on percussion. The chest X-ray shows consolidation and collapse in the affected areas. The patient should be treated aggressively with chest physiotherapy to prevent pneumonia. Patient position, regular nebulizers and deep breathing help to clear secretions and to keep the lungs fully expanded.

With elective operations, these patients can be identified preoperatively. A thoracic epidural, regular nebulizers and chest physiotherapy may help to prevent basal lung collapse.

KEY POINTS

- Patients at risk of respiratory complications should be identified preoperatively.
- Good pain control and chest physiotherapy will help prevent basal atelectasis.

CASE 97: LOW URINE OUTPUT

History

As the doctor on call you are asked to review a postoperative patient on the ward. The patient is an 86-year-old man who had a right hemicolectomy for a caecal carcinoma 2 days previously. Preoperatively, he was on antihypertensive medication which has not been restarted. During the day, his urine output had been poor with a total of 75 mL produced over the last 8 h. He has taken very little fluid orally during the day. His epidural was removed earlier that afternoon and he has been started on non-steroidal anti-inflammatory drugs (NSAIDs) for pain relief.

Examination

He is alert and orientated in time place and person. He is afebrile, blood pressure is 110/70 mmHg and pulse 110/min. His chest is clear and heart sounds are normal. His abdomen is tender around the incision, but otherwise soft and non-tender. He has normal bowel sounds and has opened his bowels since the operation.

INVESTIGATIONS

He had postoperative blood tests on day 1 which were normal. No blood tests were available from that day.

Questions

- What is normal minimal urine output expected in a 70 kg man?
- What are the causes of acute renal failure?
- What would be your approach to managing this patient?
- What biochemical changes would you see with acute renal failure?

ANSWER 97

Urine production should be greater than 0.5 mL/kg/h. The aetiology of acute renal failure can be thought of in three main categories:

- *pre-renal*: the glomerular filtration is reduced because of poor renal perfusion. This is usually caused by hypovolaemia as a result of acute blood loss, fluid depletion or hypotension. The patient's tubular and glomerular function are normal, so renal function should be restored with appropriate fluid replacement
- *renal*: this is the result of damage directly to the glomerulus or tubule. The use of drugs such as NSAIDs, contrast agents or aminoglycosides, all have direct nephrotoxic effects. Acute tubular necrosis can occur as a result of prolonged hypoperfusion, either perioperatively or postoperatively. Pre-existing renal disease such as diabetic nephropathy or glomerulonephritis makes patients more susceptible to further renal injury
- *post-renal*: this can be simply the result of a blocked catheter. This should always be checked as a cause for complete anuria in a previously fit patient. Calculi, blood clots, ureteric ligation and prostatic hypertrophy can also all lead to obstruction of urinary flow.

This patient is likely to be dehydrated as a result of his poor oral intake since his operation. Firstly, check the catheter by flushing it and palpate the abdomen for a distended bladder. Then calculate his fluid balance since the operation. Check for any evidence of sepsis. With his current blood pressure, his antihypertensive medication does not need to be restarted. It is important to maintain a good blood pressure to ensure adequate renal perfusion. The NSAIDs should be stopped as these have a direct nephrotoxic effect which may worsen his renal function.

Examine the patient for any evidence of fluid overload and check his history for previous renal problems or cardiovascular disease. Initially, the patient should be given a fluid challenge. A bolus infusion of 250 mL should give an improvement in urine output if the cause is pre-renal. If after two attempts no improvement is seen, the patient should be considered for transfer to a high-dependency unit and central-venous-pressure monitoring.

Biochemical changes in acute renal failure

- Hyponatraemia
- Hyperkalaemia
- Hypocalcaemia
- Metabolic acidosis

KEY POINT

- Urine production should be greater than 0.5 mL/kg/h.

CASE 98: VOMITING AND ABDOMINAL DISTENSION

History

You are called to the ward at 3 a.m., to see a 20-year-old man with persistent vomiting. He had an emergency laparotomy 3 days previously. The doctor on call earlier had prescribed anti-emetics for the patient, without carrying out a full assessment. The patient is extremely distressed and the nurse in charge is concerned about his sudden deterioration. You retrieve the operation note and find the patient had undergone a 'normal' laparotomy for trauma. The small and large bowel were both examined carefully and no injury was found. He had made a good recovery and had been moved onto free fluids earlier in the day. There was no nasogastric tube left after the operation, and the urinary catheter had been removed.

Examination

The patient is rolling around in the bed having just vomited. His blood pressure is 120/75 mmHg and pulse rate 110/min. He has a midline incision covered with a dry dressing. The abdomen is distended and tympanic. On palpation, he is tender around the incision only. There are no bowel sounds on auscultation.

INVESTIGATIONS

		Normal
Haemoglobin	12.0 g/dL	11.5–16.0 g/dL
Mean cell volume	82 fL	76–96 fL
White cell count	10.2×10^9/L	$4.0–11.0 \times 10^9$/L
Platelets	253×10^9/L	$150–400 \times 10^9$/L
Sodium	132 mmol/L	135–145 mmol/L
Potassium	2.9 mmol/L	3.5–5.0 mmol/L
Urea	5.0 mmol/L	2.5–6.7 mmmol/L
Creatinine	54 μmol/L	44–80 μmol/L

An X-ray of the abdomen is shown in Fig. 98.1.

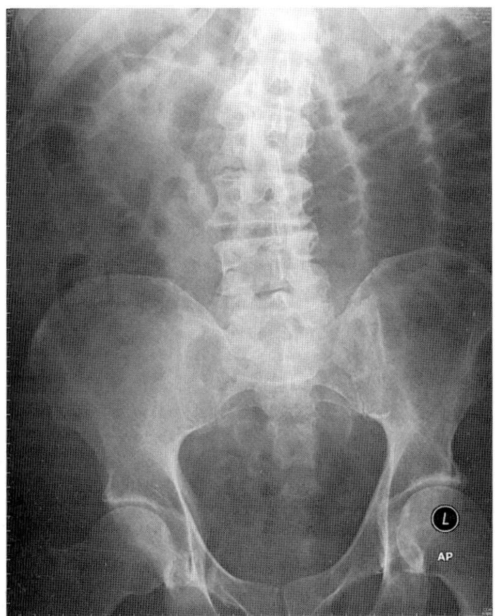

Figure 98.1 Plain X-ray of the abdomen.

Questions

- What is shown on the abdominal X-ray?
- What are the most common causes?
- What is the most likely cause in this patient?
- How would you manage the patient?

ANSWER 98

When assessing a postoperative patient on the ward it is important to read the operation note as well as making a physical assessment. Unexpected findings or difficulties during the procedure should be documented, and this may aid your clinical decision making. This patient has a postoperative paralytic ileus. An ileus is a normal physiological event after abdominal surgery. It usually resolves spontaneously within 2–3 days of the procedure. Paralytic ileus is defined as ileus of the intestine persisting for more than 3 days after surgery. His bowels had not returned to normal function by day 3 and he had started free fluids that morning. This resulted in vomiting and abdominal discomfort.

A nasogastric tube should be placed to decompress the bowel, and a urinary catheter inserted to monitor his urine output. Non-steroidal anti-inflammatory drugs (NSAIDs) can be used for pain relief, rather than opiates, as these will not affect bowel motility.

The most common cause of an ileus is an intra-abdominal operation. Other factors can prolong an ileus and should be looked for and corrected if possible. This patient has hypokalaemia which should be corrected.

! Causes of ileus

- *Sepsis*: intra-abdominal inflammation and peritonitis
- *Drugs*: opioids, antacids
- *Metabolic*: hypokalaemia, hyponatraemia, hypomagnesia, anaemia
- *Myocardial infarction*
- *Pneumonia*
- *Head injury and neurosurgical procedures*
- *Retroperitoneal haematomas*

For patients with protracted ileus, mechanical obstruction should be excluded by a small-bowel follow through or a computerized tomography scan. Before further investigation, underlying sepsis or electrolyte abnormalities should be corrected. Medications that produce ileus (e.g. opiates) should also be stopped.

KEY POINTS

- Postoperative ileus should resolve after 2–3 days.
- Electrolyte abnormalities are a common cause of paralytic ileus during the postoperative period.

CASE 99: SUDDEN SHORTNESS OF BREATH

History

As the doctor on call, you are asked to see a 66-year-old woman on the orthopaedic ward who has become acutely short of breath. She is 7 days post hemiarthroplasty for a fractured femur and her recovery has been slow. When you arrive the patient has an oxygen mask on and is feeling more comfortable. She is still complaining of pain on deep inspiration and finds it difficult to talk in full sentences. She has no known cardiovascular disease, but is overweight. She is an ex-smoker.

Examination

The patient is tachypnoeic with a respiratory rate of 35/min and oxygen saturations of 92 per cent on 35 per cent oxygen. She is afebrile and has a blood pressure of 100/80 mmHg and a pulse rate of 120/min. There is good air entry throughout on both sides of the chest. Abdominal examination is unremarkable.

INVESTIGATIONS

		Normal
Haemoglobin	13.0 g/dL	11.5–16.0 g/dL
Mean cell volume	84 fL	76–96 fL
White cell count	11.2×10^9/L	$4.0–11.0 \times 10^9$/L
Platelets	235×10^9/L	$150–400 \times 10^9$/L
Sodium	135 mmol/L	135–145 mmol/L
Potassium	4.0 mmol/L	3.5–5.0 mmol/L
Urea	6.0 mmol/L	2.5–6.7 mmmol/L
Creatinine	55 μmol/L	44–80 μmol/L
pH	7.38	7.36–7.44
Partial pressure of CO_2 (pCO_2)	3.8 kPa	4.7–5.9 kPa
Partial pressure of O_2 (pO_2)	6.6 kPa	11–13 kPa
Base excess	–1.1	±2)
Lactate	1.0	<2 mmol/L

Figure 99.1 shows an electrocardiogram (ECG).

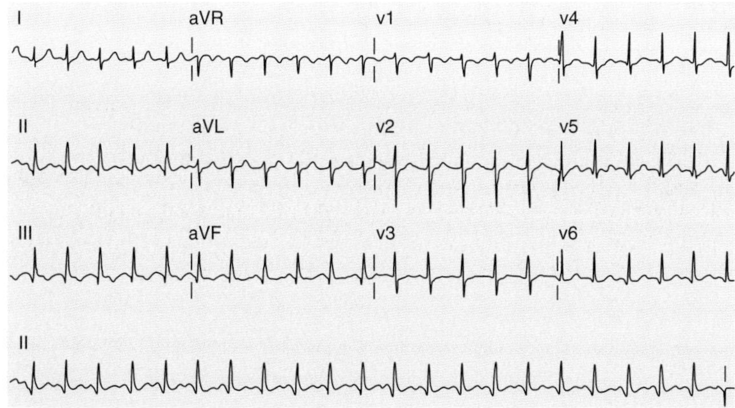

Figure 99.1 Electrocardiogram.

Questions

- What is the likely diagnosis?
- What are the risk factors?
- How would you treat the patient?
- Which investigations would confirm your diagnosis?

ANSWER 99

The patient has had a pulmonary embolism (PE). The sudden shortness of breath, pleuritic chest pain, recent lower-limb surgery and drop in po_2 support this diagnosis. The ECG shows a S1 Q3 T3 anomaly which is consistent with right heart strain due caused by a large obstructing embolus. These ECG changes are not always seen, the commonest findings being either a normal ECG or a sinus tachycardia.

! Risk factors for pulmonary embolism

- Surgery and trauma
- Hypercoagulable states
- Pregnancy
- Oral contraceptives and oestrogen replacement
- Malignancy
- Stroke
- Indwelling venous catheters
- Previous history/family history of venous thromboembolism
- Congestive heart failure
- Obesity

The risk of pulmonary embolism increases with prolonged bed rest or immobilization. Pulmonary emboli usually arise from thrombi originating in the deep venous system of the lower extremities, but may originate in the pelvic, renal, or upper extremity veins and the right heart chambers. The patient should be placed on high-flow oxygen and arterial blood gases should be taken. A chest X-ray is required to exclude other pathology. If clinical suspicion is high the patient should be anticoagulated with low-molecular-weight heparin until the diagnosis is confirmed with either a $\dot{V}/\dot{Q}$ (ventilation–perfusion) scan or a CT pulmonary angiogram. A duplex scan of the lower limbs may confirm the origin of the embolus. The patient should then be started on long-term warfarin provided there are no contraindications.

KEY POINTS

- All surgical patients require prophylactic heparin to prevent deep vein thrombosis.
- If a PE is suspected, anticoagulation should be started prior to confirmation of the diagnosis.

CASE 100: POSTOPERATIVE SEPSIS

History

You are asked to review a 67-year-old man on the orthopaedic ward who underwent a total knee replacement 4 days ago. The nursing staff report that he has developed a temperature over the last 24 h. He was making a good postoperative recovery and had his urinary catheter removed 48 h ago. He reports no chest symptoms. He is eating and drinking and has opened his bowels normally. He passed urine 2 h ago. His past medical history includes hypertension and depression. He takes ramipril 5 mg od, simvastatin 40 mg and sertraline 50 mg od. Up until 3 years ago he smoked 20 cigarettes a day. He does not drink alcohol. He is married and is a retired accountant.

Examination

He has a temperature of 37.8°C with a pulse rate of 92/min and a blood pressure of 114/82 mmHg. The oxygen saturations are 96 per cent on room air. He is comfortable in bed but looks flushed. He is orientated in time, place and person. His cardiorespiratory and abdominal examinations are unremarkable. He has no calf swelling or tenderness. The wound looks dry and the knee has a typical postoperative appearance.

INVESTIGATIONS

		Normal
Haemoglobin	11.8 g/dL	11.5–16.0 g/dL
Mean cell volume	86 fL	76–96 fL
White cell count (WCC)	15.6×10^9/L	$4.0–11.0 \times 10^9$/L
Platelets	289×10^9/L	$150–400 \times 10^9$/L
Erythrocyte sedimentation rate (ESR)	34 mm/h	10–20 mm/h
Sodium	135 mmol/L	135–145 mmol/L
Potassium	3.9 mmol/L	3.5–5.0 mmol/L
Urea	5.1 mmol/L	2.5–6.7 mmmol/L
Creatinine	78 μmol/L	44–80 μmol/L
C-reactive protein (CRP)	88 mg/L	<5 mg/L

D-dimer: positive

Urinalysis

WCC: +++

Protein: ++

Nitrite: positive

Blood: +

Electrocardiogram (ECG): normal

Questions

- What tests form the basis of a 'septic screen'?
- What is the likely diagnosis?
- How should he be managed?

ANSWER 100

It is very common to be called to see a postoperative patient with a raised temperature. In the first 24 h after the operation a temperature rise may occur as a result of the release of inflammatory mediators from traumatized tissues. Temperatures occuring after 24 h are commonly due to pneumonia, urinary tract infection, wound infection, deep vein thrombosis, pulmonary embolism, bowel obstruction or ileus. With this in mind, after completing a full history and examination, a 'septic screen' should be performed.

! Septic screen

- Urine dipstick and urine sent for microscopy, culture and sensitivity
- Blood cultures
- Sputum cultures
- Wound swab – if appropriate
- Chest X-ray

Other useful tests that should also be performed are:

- full blood count/urea and electrolytes/C-reactive protein
- ECG: useful to exclude a cardiac cause
- arterial blood gases: if septic or hypoxic.

In this case, the patient has developed a urinary tract infection; the clues in the scenario are the history of previous catheterization and the urine dipstick positive for both nitrites and leucocytes. The D-dimer test should be interpreted with caution as it invariably goes up after surgery. Similarly, because of their lack of specificity, CRP and ESR are of limited value. Empirical antibiotic treatment should be commenced after the urine is sent for culture and sensitivity. The presence of a bacteraemia could lead to a potentially devastating infection of the knee prosthesis, so in this patient there is an argument for giving the initial doses of antibiotics intravenously, to ensure that high tissue levels are reached quickly.

KEY POINT

- A septic screen should be done to investigate the cause of a postoperative pyrexia.

INDEX

References are by case number with relevant page number(s) following in brackets. References with a page range e.g. 25(68–70) indicate that although the subject may be mentioned only on one page, it concerns the whole case.